W9-ARQ-932

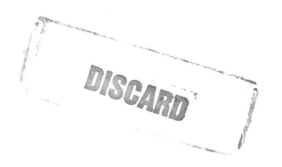

Springer

Tokyo
Berlin
Heidelberg
New York
Hong Kong
London
Milan
Paris

Recent Advances in Endourology, 4

S. Ohshima, Y. Hirao (Eds.)

Clinical Guidelines in Urological Management

With 16 Figures

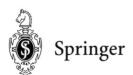 Springer

Shinichi Ohshima, M.D., Ph.D.
Vice-President
Nagoya University Hospital
Professor and Chairman
Department of Urology
Nagoya University Graduate School of Medicine
65 Tsurumai-cho, Showa-ku, Nagoya 466-8550, Japan

Yoshihiko Hirao, M.D.
Professor and Chairman
Department of Urology
Nara Prefectural Medical University
840 Shijo-cho, Kashihara, Nara 634-0813, Japan

ISBN 4-431-70342-X Springer-Verlag Tokyo Berlin Heidelberg New York

Library of Congress Cataloging-in-Publication Data

Clinical guidelines in urological management / S. Ohshima, Y. Hirao, eds.
        p. ; cm.—(Recent advances in endourology ; 4)
    Includes bibliographical references and index.
    ISBN 443170342X (hardcover : alk. paper)
    1. Urology—Practice. 2. Medical protocols. I. Ohshima, S. (Shinichi), 1945– II. Hirao,
Y. (Yoshihiko), 1947– III. Series.
    [DNLM: 1. Practice Guidelines. 2. Urologic Diseases—therapy. WJ 140 C64025 2003]
RC872 .C56 2003
616.6—dc21

                                                                    2002030505

Printed on acid-free paper

Typesetting: SNP Best-set Typesetter Ltd., Hong Kong
Printing and binding: Shinano, Incorporated, Japan
SPIN: 10886212 series number 4130

Foreword

The twenty-first century will be the era of the market economy, a century characterized by the penetration of market forces into every social field, even into government activities, education, and medical care.

Guidelines for the provision of clinical care have been developed in recent years chiefly in American health-care services, which are the most thoroughly exposed to the market economy. The problem of escalating medical costs in the United States led the government and consumer groups to introduce clinical practice guidelines. Guidelines were introduced to control medical costs and quality. Initially, guidelines were developed mainly on the consumer side, but professionals, too, soon recognized the importance of clinical practice guidelines. The involvement of diverse groups in the development of guidelines has intensified the need to create and improve scientific methods for drawing up those guidelines.

Owing to the development of systematic and structured abstraction methods, evidence-based guidelines have been proposed. Principally, guidelines are a summary of published treatments created by statistical analysis of clinical outcomes. The method of summarizing outcomes of different treatment procedures is statistical meta-analysis. Therefore, the findings inevitably depend on the published findings. The limitations of meta-analysis exist in the source of information rather than in the methods utilized. Science-based guidelines serve to improve the quality of clinical care and its assessment, and to reduce the financial costs of inappropriate care. The conflict between the payer, consumer, and practitioner cannot be resolved by guidelines, but guidelines are rational social judgments about what care should be covered by public and private health-care plans.

In Japan, the medical insurance and reimbursement system is tightly controlled by the government bureaucracy and is not directly exposed to the market economy. The government creates Clinical Practice Reimbursement Guidelines (CPRGs), which are not based on an evidence-based scientific approach but on bureaucrats' opinions from the standpoints of rationalizing budgets and preventing inappropriate use of medical care. Professionals and medical groups express opinions about the content of CPRGs, but their opinions are mostly ignored.

Generally, clinical practice guidelines, unlike CPRGs, are not synonymous with reimbursement or coverage policies. However, the CPRG system may, hopefully speaking, be constructed in a manner compatible with science-based guidelines. This book is published in the hope that medical reimbursement policies will depend not only on budget rationalization but also on scientific guidelines.

E. Higashihara, M.D.
President, Japanese Society of Endourology and ESWL
Professor and Chairman, Department of Urology
Kyorin University School of Medicine

Preface

In recent years, standardization of clinical practices has been required, both to improve the quality of those practices and to establish a more efficient system of costs for medical practices. Guidelines for clinical practice, developed from evidence-based medicine by a panel of physicians, surgeons, and other medical professionals, clearly can lead to better diagnostic procedures and treatment modalities for patients.

In clinical practice, decision making usually proceeds by hearing patients' complaints, considering the findings of physical examinations, and reviewing laboratory, radiology, and ultrasonography data. The clinical experience of individual doctors also contributes. However, as a result of the rapid development of diagnostic procedures and treatment modalities, too many articles are published for us to use them effectively. We benefit, therefore, by having new information summarized for us. That is one reason why clinical practice guidelines are required.

Another reason for guidelines is that in the 1970s, clinical practice changed in a revolutionary manner, from paternalism to partnership. The main concepts of a partnership between patients and clinicians are informed consent and patients' self-determination. Previously, the principles of medical practice were an issue between individual doctors, but they now have become a social issue. Now, not only disclosure of medical information but also accountability to society is called for. As professionals in the field of medicine, clinicians have a responsibility to explain the standard treatment modality based on scientific evidence. It is therefore a great pleasure to participate in this review of clinical practice guidelines in the field of urology.

Shinichi Ohshima, M.D., Ph.D.
Vice-President, Nagoya University Hospital
Professor and Chairman, Department of Urology
Nagoya University Graduate School of Medicine

Contents

Contributors

Developing Clinical Practice Guidelines

KIERAN J. O'FLYNN

Summary. Clinical practice guidelines are systematically developed statements to assist decision-making on appropriate health care for specific clinical circumstances. The primary objective of a clinical guideline is to improve the quality of clinical care by making evidence-based advice on best practice available to health care professionals and patients. Good clinical guidelines will need to take into account the effect on stakeholders and relevant factors in the local delivery of health care. Guidelines require a rigorous review and analysis of peer-reviewed research. Ideally, the guideline should be firmly based on reliable evidence of clinical and cost-effectiveness. An integral part of guideline development is the need to identify the potential barriers that may prevent its successful implementation. An active educational intervention should be considered to enable effective dissemination of the guideline. As new knowledge emerges, guidelines may quickly becouse out of date, and arrangements should be put in place to reassess the validity of the guideline at some point in the future.

Key Words. Guidelines, Critical appraisal, Evidence, Development, Implementation

Introduction

For many clinicians, one of the biggest obstacles to practicing effectively is the explosion in medical knowledge, which has led to an exponential growth in the volume of medical literature. There are approximately 3–4 million new biomedical publications per year in over 20000 journals, and it has been estimated that the sum of medical knowledge doubles every 19 years [1]. The volume of literature and the limited time and resources means that many clinicians have difficulty keeping up to date with recent advances in their field. The introduction of

Department of Urology, Hope Hospital, Eccles Old Road, Salford, Greater Manchester M6 8HD, UK clinical guidelines is seen increasingly as a means of improving health care outcomes and reducing costs.

Clinical practice guidelines have been defined by the US Institute of Medicine as "systematically developed statements to assist practitioner and patient on decisions about appropriate health care for specific clinical circumstances" [2]. They represent an attempt to distill a large volume of medical literature into a convenient, usable form, making explicit recommendations with a definite intention of influencing what clinicians do.

Guidelines can be used in a wide variety of settings to promote effective and efficient health care. Guidelines may encompass a number of health care interventions, for example, the introduction of a new procedure or service on the promotion of effective health care in a primary or secondary setting, or to encourage the adoption of cost-effective interventions. The primary objective of a clinical guideline is to improve the quality of clinical care by making evidence-based advice on best practice available to health care professionals and patients.

Getting Started

Central to the issue of a clinical guideline is the precise definition of the clinical issue to be addressed. This issue is crucial, became a precise definition may convert an unwieldy global problem into a number of smaller ones. For example, generating clinical policies for the evaluation and treatment of men with prostate cancer is much more difficult than generating guidelines for specific subgroups of men within this large population. It seems sensible to develop guidelines on clinical topics for which the evidence is robust and generally noncontroversial, yet for which evidence exists that the condition is not being managed appropriately.

A key element in the development of a successful guideline is forming the right team. The process of formulating a guideline will go through a number of separate stages, from the issues to be addressed by the guideline, through identifying the relevant evidence, distilling it into a usable form, and disseminating the guideline to relevant health care practitioners. Care paid to each of these steps is more likely to result in implementation of the guideline and, hopefully, an improvement in clinical care.

The team will need to have a variety of skills, such as ability to contribute to the clinical discussion, people with training skills, and those who can influence the deployment of resources. It is vitally important to identify all the clinicians, nurses, managers, patient representatives, and others who may be affected by a new clinical guideline. Getting the right team to develop the guideline should help enormously in the identification of individual and organizational barriers to the implementation of the guideline, allowing specific strategies to be identified and budgetary restraints to be overcome.

Representatives of all the stakeholders potentially affected by the introduction of a new guideline should be identified and actively engaged in the process.

Patients can be strong advocates for change and may provide valuable insights into the proposed changes. Local ownership of a guideline is likely to result in less negative feedback when efforts are being made to implement the new guideline.

The Process of Developing a New Clinical Guideline

The best guidelines will provide a description of the sources of information used to identify and select the evidence on which the guidelines are based [3]. Guideline developers must bring together all the relevant evidence and combine that evidence in an appropriate manner. This necessitates converting the clinical information required into answerable questions, tracking down the best evidence with which to answer them, and a careful examination of the validity (closeness to the truth) and usefulness (clinical applicability) of the identified publications [4]. Each publication can then be graded (see Table 1) in an objective way, allowing for the development of consensus among the authors of the guideline about what recommendations to endorse.

Certain study designs are superior to others for answering particular questions. Randomized controlled trials (RCTs) are considered by many the gold standard for addressing questions regarding therapeutic efficacy. Ideally the best guidelines would draw on systematic reviews and randomized controlled trials, which link specific interventions with outcome. Unfortunately, many important clinical problems are technically, economically, or ethically difficult to address with randomized controlled trials. Consequently, developers of clinical guidelines will frequently deal with different types of evidence, including not only systematic reviews, meta-analyses, a variety of controlled trials, but also case-control and cohort studies, which are appropriate for addressing questions related to etiology or risk. The evidence will need to be supplemented with the advice of experts and the experience of clinicians and patients.

A good starting point in developing a guideline is a review produced by a reputable source. However, reviews are frequently written by experts in their field and tend to be selective in their appraisal of the current literature and may generate incorrect conclusions and inappropriate or harmful clinical recommendations [5]. A systematic review is an overview of primary studies that uses explicit and reproducible methods [6]. A close examination of systematic reviews of primary studies that use an explicit and reproducible methodology is an essential first step in the development of a clinical guideline. A meta-analysis is a mathematical synthesis of the results of two or more primary studies that address the same hypothesis in the same way. The rationale for systematic reviews and meta-analysis is based on a number of premises. First, given the huge volume of literature, information on a particular topic must be reduced to easily digestible pieces. The systematic review should separate information that is salient and critical from that which is unsound, anecdotal, or simply biased. In a good-quality systematic review the question(s) to be answered and the methods used will be

TABLE 1. Levels of evidence and grades of recommendations[a]

Grade of recommendation	Level	Therapy/prevention etiology/harm	Prognosis	Diagnosis	Differential diagnosis symptom prevalence study	Economic and decision analysis
A	1a	Systematic review with homogeneity of RCTs	Systematic review with homogeneity of inception cohort studies	Systematic review of level 1 diagnostic studies	Systematic review of prospective cohort studies	Systematic review with homogeneity of level 1 economic studies
	1b	Individual RCT (with narrow confidence interval)	Individual inception cohort study with >80% follow-up	Validating study with good reference standards	Prospective cohort study with >80% follow-up over adequate period	Systematic review of evidence
B	2a	Systematic review with homogeneity of cohort studies	Systematic review with homgeneity of cohort study or follow-up of untreated control patients in RCT	Systematic review with homogeneity of level >2 diagnostic studies	Systematic review with homogeneity of level 2b and better studies	Systematic review with homogeneity of level >2 economic studies
	2b	Individual cohort study or low-quality RCT <80% follow-up	Retrospective cohort study or follow-up of untreated control patients in RCT	Exploratory cohort study with good reference standards	Retrospective cohort study, or poor follow-up	Analysis based on clinically sensible costs or alternatives; limited reviews
	3a	Systematic review with homgeneity of case-control studies		Systematic review with homogeneity of 3b and better studies	Systematic review with homogeneity of of 3b and better studies	Systematic review with homogeneity of 3b and better studies
	3b	Individual case-control study		Nonconsecutive study or without consistently applied reference standards	Nonconsecutive cohort study or very limited population	Analysis based on limited alternatives or costs, but includes sensitivity analysis
C	4	Case series (and poor-quality cohort and case-control studies)	Case series (and poor quality prognostic cohort studies	Case-control study or nonindependent reference standard	Case series	Analysis with no sensitivity analysis
D	5	Expert opinion without explicit critical appraisal or based on "first principles"	Expert opinion without explicit critical appraisal or based on "first principles"	Expert opinion without explicit critical appraisal or based on "first principles"	Expert opinion without explicit critical appraisal or based on "first principles"	Expert opinion without explicit critical appraisal or based on "first principles"

RCT, randomized controlled trial.

[a] Adapted from the Oxford Centre for Evidence-Based Medicine Levels of Evidence (May 2001).

Reference: http://cebm.jr2.ox.ac.uk/docs/levels.html.

clearly stated. Every effort will have been made to identify all relevant studies, published or not. This is particularly important, because submitted studies with negative results are less likely to get published, and this may result in bias.

Potentially randomized controlled trials provide the best evidence we can obtain about causation (whether it concerns etiology, therapeutics, or the role of new surgical procedures). The aim of randomization is to avoid selection bias and to generate groups that are comparable to each other. In reviewing a randomized controlled trial to support the development of a clinical guideline, the reviewer must be satisfied that a number of criteria have been met [4]. These include no foreknowledge of patient allocation to a particular treatment arm, no bias in patient management, no bias in the outcome assessment of the patient, and an intention-to-treat analysis of the data, with no post-randomization exclusions.

Case series abound in the urological literature, and it is imperative that developers of guidelines be aware of their strengths and weaknesses. Many medical or surgical interventions cannot be evaluated by a randomized controlled trial. Carefully performed observational studies provide valuable information on clinical outcome, and they may show clinical uncertainty, generate a new hypothesis, or modify and refine a new surgical technique. Some therapeutic interventions have an impact so large that observational data alone are sufficient to show an outcome benefit, as evidenced by the introduction of extraconpored shock-wave lithotripsy (ESWL) for renal calculi. Unlike randomized controlled trials, which usually run for a fixed period of time and may fail to detect infrequent adverse outcomes, observational data provide a realistic means of assessing the long-term outcome of a new medicine or surgical intervention. Careful observation and reporting of the evaluation of a new surgical procedure is valid evidence. However, developers of clinical guidelines need to be aware that case series provide the weakest evidence for assessing the efficacy of a treatment, because they are subject to uncontrolled biases, particularly in patient selection. In assessing the results of observational studies, developers of clinical guidelines may find it appropriate to conduct sensitivity analyses to determine the implications if the results of the observational studies represented overestimates or underestimates of the true effect of the intervention on the relevant outcome.

Even in the presence of strong evidence from randomized clinical trials, the size effect of the intervention may be small or the intervention may be associated with costs, side effects, or impracticalities that may lead to disagreement among guideline developers about what management to recommend. The guideline will reflect a value judgment about the relative importance of various health and economic outcomes in a specific clinical situation. The guideline developers will need to consider not only the best management options, but also all the important consequences of the options.

It is sensible to avoid spending too much time looking for the right evidence. It is relatively easy to identify new publications through careful and methodical Medline searches, but interpreting them carefully may take a lot of effort. The evidence base is continually evolving, and extra time and resources might be better spent on persuading clinicians to change their practice during the implementation phase of the guideline.

Converting the Evidence into Clinical Policy

An effective guideline is written with the expressed intention of influencing what clinicians do in a specific clinical situation. The suggestions about how a particular condition will be managed will go beyond a simple presentation of evidence, costs, and decision models. A guideline will reflect value judgments (made by the agency responsible for the guideline) of various health and economic outcomes in specific clinical situations and will need to reflect the real-world situation of the reader of the guideline. A good guideline will have a description of the methods used to formulate recommendations and will give explicit information about the strength of the evidence and the degree of consensus in the recommendations [7].

The strength of a guideline recommendation should be informed by a number of considerations: the quality of the investigations appraised for the recommendations, the magnitude and consistency of positive outcomes compared with negative outcomes, and the relative value placed on outcomes. Although there may be strong evidence from randomized clinical trials, the overall size effect may be small, and the intervention may be associated with costs, side effects, or practical implications that will reduce the strength of the recommendation about what clinicians should do.

What can go wrong? Guideline development groups often lack the time, resources, and skills to scrutinize the evidence in detail. Frequently there is insufficient or misleading scientific information about what to recommend, and the value judgments made by a guideline group may be the wrong choice for individual patients. Recommendations made by guideline committees are influenced by opinions, clinical experience, the composition of the group, and the uncertainties of group dynamics.

Implementation of the Clinical Guideline

Implementation is possibly the most important component of a successful clinical guideline. Careful consideration should be given to the knock –on effect of the introduction of a new guideline. There is little point in persuading clinicians to change their practice if the service cannot cope with the extra demand. For this reason, it is prudent to carefully think through the implications of the guideline before the guideline is disseminated.

There is, unfortunately, no evidence that merely circulating a clinical guideline will result in a change in clinical practice [8], although this method may be useful in raising awareness of a particular issue. In the UK, organizations such as the National Institute of Clinical Excellence (NICE) and the NHS Centre for

TABLE 2. Useful sources of information on the Internet for developing guidelines

Resource	Website	Comment
American College of Physicians online	http://www.acponline.org/	Allows access to ACP journal club and Evidence-Based Medicine
National Institutes of Health	http://www.nih.gov	Publications and fact sheets on a wide variety of topics with A-Z topic index, database of clinical trials. Allows access to information on the NIH Consensus Development Program, the focal point for evidence-based assessments of medical practice
The Cochrane Collaboration	http://www.cochrane.org/	This site contains detailed information on the Cochrane Centres, the collaborative review groups, register of RCTs, and systematic reviews, and detailed bibliographies on many evidence-based medicine issues
NHS Centre for Reviews and Dissemination	http://www.york.ac.uk/inst/crd/welcome.htm	A rapidly expanding database of systematic reviews concerned with the effectiveness of health care interventions
Centre for Evidence-Based Medicine	http://cebm.jr2.ox.ac.uk	This site has a wealth of information on evidence-based medicine terms and provides useful information and links on critical appraisal
Oncolink (University of Pennysylvania Cancer Center)	http://cancer.med.upenn.edu/resources/	Detailed information on all aspects of cancer. All trials being conducted by the National Cancer Institute are cited and discussed

Reviews and Dissemination (see Table 2) are leading an increased tendency to formulate and disseminate national guidance throughout the National Health Service. The performance of systematic reviews of therapy has become the focus of a rapidly growing international group of clinicians, epidemiologists, and consumers, who have formed the Cochrane Collaboration. All of these resources can be easily accessed over the Internet (see Table 2).

Altering physicians' clinical practice will depend on the extent to which the message can be got across to busy clinicians. A new guideline is unlikely to be successful if effective training and education are not organized for clinical staff. For many common conditions, this requires the close collaboration of primary and secondary health care professionals.

A number of different interventions can be tried to gain greater acceptance of a new clinical guideline. Most interventions are effective under some circumstances, but none are effective under all circumstances. Evidence from North America suggests that using a trained professional to meet with health care professionals in their practice setting and providing information on a particular topic may alter clinical practice [9]. Using reminder systems is usually effective for a range of behaviors. Good evidence on the use of local opinion leaders to alter clinical practice is lacking, although this approach is frequently used [10]. Guidelines are frequently bulky documents, and distilling the salient information into algorithms and flow charts may be beneficial in getting the message across. In general, multifaceted interventions targeting different barriers to change are more likely to be effective than single interventions [8].

The key challenge in the successful dissemination of a guideline is to persuade clinicians of the value of the evidence so that they can decide whether the guideline may help the process of patient care. Guidelines are advisory documents, and individual physicians will have different perception of risks and tradeoffs in a given clinical situation. In addition, the clinician will need to take into account the patient's understanding, beliefs, and preferences about what course of action to take [7]. Some clinicians do not have a scientific perspective or framework for decision-making, and they may weight their personal experiences more heavily than the information derived from a guideline. Targeting clinicians known to be resistant to change may help promote the successful implementation of the guideline.

The long-term goal of a clinical guideline is to ensure that there is an improvement in the quality of care provided to the patient. Playing close attention to practical considerations may help. Creating reminder systems as part of a patient's record may help. Ongoing induction training for new staff will continue to promote the change.

Evaluation and Feedback

Research findings on altering professional behavior indicate that dissemination activities are relatively ineffective in directly changing clinical practice [8]. After all the hard work of developing a guideline, it is worthwhile assessing the impact of the guidance on clinical care. In addition, the introduction of a clinical guideline provides a standard against which health professionals can monitor their own clinical practice by audit. Audit and feedback can be effective in improving performance, in particular in test ordering and prescribing, although the effects are generally small to moderate [11]. Exploration of the issues behind the success or

- A clear, concise statement of the clinical practice to be addressed
- Identifying the right team
- Finding and appraising the evidence
- Converting the evidence into clinical policy
- Disseminating the clinical guideline

FIG. 1. Key steps in the development of a clinical practice guideline

- Applicability—Are the patients (and clinicians) for whom the guideline is intended clearly identified? Is there a description of circumstances in which exceptions might be made in using the guidelines?
- Representative—Should involve key groups of health care practitioners and patient representatives
- Validity—Were the guidelines subjected to independent review by experts prior to publication or release?
- Reproducibility—If others appraised the same evidence, would they come to the same result?
- Cost-effective—Make appropriate use of resources
- Clarity—Easily understood by clinicians and patients
- Updating—Is there mention of a date for reviewing or updating the guideline?
- Amenable to clinical audit

FIG. 2. What makes a good clinical guideline?

failure of a newly implemented guideline may ultimately help other colleagues learn from the endeavors of the development team.

Conclusion

The development of evidence-based guidelines holds considerable promise for continued improvement in the delivery of health care. Good clinical guidelines should consider all the relevant disciplines and stakeholders and will have to take into account relevant factors in the local delivery of health care. Guidelines require a rigorous review and analysis of peer-reviewed research and should in turn be subjected to peer review. They should be firmly based on reliable evi-

- **Are the results valid?**

  Were all important options and outcomes specified?

  Was there an explicit and sensible process used to identify and appraise the evidence?

  Was there an explicit and sensible process used to consider the relative values of different outcomes?

  Were important recent developments included?

  Has the guideline been peer reviewed and tested?

- **What are the recommendations?**

  How strong are the recommendations?

  Are the recommendations practical?

- **Will the results help in patient care?**

  Do I share similar objectives with the guidelines?

  Are the recommendations applicable to my patients?

Fig. 3. Using a clinical practice guideline

dence of clinical and cost-effectiveness. Any systematic approach to changing clinical behavior by the introduction of a guideline needs to identify the potential barriers to change and include an active educational intervention to enable effective dissemination of the results. Guidelines frequently address controversial health issues, about which new knowledge is actively sought in new studies, and consequently they may quickly become dated. Arrangements should be put in place to reassess the validity of the guideline at some point in the future.

References

1. Smith R (1996) What information do doctors need? BMJ 313:1062–1068
2. Institute of Medicine. Field MJ, Lohr KN (eds) (1990) Clinical practice guidelines: directions for a new program. National Academy Press, Washington, DC
3. Wilson MC, Hayward RSA, Tunis SR, Bass EB, Guyatt G (1995) User's guides to the medical literature. VIII. How to use clinical practice guidelines. A. Are the recommendations valid? JAMA 274:57–574
4. Sackett DL, Richardson WC, Rosenberg W, Haynes RB (1997) Evidence based medicine. How to practise and teach EBM. Churchill Livingstone, New York

5. Antman EM, Lau J, et al. (1992) A comparsion of results of meta-analyses of ran-domized control trials and recommendations of clinical experts. JAMA 268:240–248
6. Mulrow CD (1995) Rationale for systematic reviews. In: Chalmers I, Altman DG (eds) Systematic reviews. BMJ Publishing Group, pp. 1–9
7. Wilson MC, Hayward RSA, Tunis SR, Bass EB, Guyatt G (1995) Users' guides to the medical literature. VIII. How to use clinical practice guidelines. B. What are the results and will they help me in caring for my patients? JAMA 274:1630–1632
8. NHS Centre for Reviews and Dissemination (1999) Effective health care. Getting evidence into practice. 1999.5(1)
9. Thomson MA, Oxman AD, Haynes RB, Freemantle N, Harvey EI (1999) Outreach visits to improve health professional practice and health care outcomes (Cochrane Review). In: The Cochrane Library, Issue 1. Oxford Update Software
10. Thomson MA, Oxman AD, Haynes RB, Freemantle N, Harvey EI (1999) Local opinion leaders to improve health professional practice and health care outcomes (Cochrane Review). In: The Cochrane Library, Issue 1. Oxford Update Software
11. Thomson MA, Oxman AD, Haynes RB, Freemantle N, Harvey EI (1999) Audit and feedback to improve health professional practice and health care outcomes (Cochrane Review). In: The Cochrane Library, Issue 1. Oxford Update Software

Evaluation of Clinical Practice Guidelines

TOMONORI HASEGAWA

Summary. Evidence-based medicine is a process approach to secure a standardized and optimal medical intervention for a given disease state based on a certain methodology. The results of evidence-based medicine activities are usually expressed as clinical practice guidelines (CPGs). CPGs should be evaluated at three different levels: the validity in selecting the disease, the validity of the CPG development process, and the impact of CPGs on medicine. Validity in selecting the disease means that it is justified to invest resources to develop the CPG for the disease. The disease will be prioritized and it will be regarded as worth investing resources to develop the CPG for the disease if: medical interventions by physicians vary, a new effective medical intervention that has been developed is not used widely, the disease affects many patients or has high costs of treatment, or the disease imposes a high risk on patients. A CPG should be developed by proper processes, and validated by other persons later. Validity, reliability and reproducibility, clinical applicability, clinical flexibility, clarity, a multidisciplinary process, scheduled review, and documentation are required for good CPGs. CPGs can change two criteria for evaluating the quality of health care, process and outcome, in two directions: standardization and improvement. Showing the impact of CPGs takes a great effort and is difficult to do, and only limited reports are available. Evidence-based medicine is an effective tool, but it is a process approach and the impact of the process approach should be measured using a highly useful standard: the outcome.

Key Words. Evaluation, Evidence-based medicine, Process approach, Clinical practice guideline, Standardization

Department of Public Health, Toho University School of Medicine, 5-21-16 Omori-nishi, Ota-ku, Tokyo 143-8540, Japan

Guideline Development Using an Evidence-Based Method

Evidence-based medicine is a process approach to secure a standardized and optimal medical intervention for a given disease state based on a certain methodology. The results of evidence-based medicine activities are usually expressed as clinical practice guidelines (CPGs). Evidence-based guideline development uses a certain methodology that was originally derived from clinical epidemiology and other academic fields, such as clinical decision-making and health economics.

To evaluate CPGs, the key steps by which the CPGs are developed must be reviewed. For details of developing the CPGs, see the chapter 6 by O'Flynn in this volume. A CPG is developed though the steps described below.

1. Selection of Disease

Because CPG development requires resources, such as manpower and money, priority setting is mandatory. Diseases are prioritized based on the following criteria:

- Medical interventions by physicians vary
- A new effective medical intervention has been developed but is not used widely
- The disease affects many patients, has a high cost of treatment, or imposes a high risk (mortality or disability) on patients

A CPG is developed to recommend standardized and optimal medical interventions for a patient with a given disease. The CPG can contribute quality to health care by specifying a certain intervention as optimal. If every physician uses the same intervention, the intervention should be regarded as a standard, and the CPG will be of no use. The burden of a disease can be estimated by using statistics such as numbers of patients and admissions, health care expenditures, and causes of death. In developed countries, such statistics are usually available, but finding and compiling them to evaluate the burden of the disease is sometimes difficult, because they are fragmented and are kept separately in various ministries and organizations. Legislation for protection of privacy sometimes makes the situation more complex. In Japan, although no legislation exists for the protection of individual health-related information, a bill currently under discussion known as the Individual Information Protection Law, will limit the linking of fragmented individual information by the use of identification codes, such as social security number and telephone number.

2. Standard Patient

A standard patient is defined as a typical patient with a disease that is the target of the CPG. No definite rule exists for how to cope with a standard patient, but such patients need profound consideration and a touch of common sense. If the standard patient concept covers too wide a range of patients with a disease, the CPG will be complex and large in volume, and because a long time is needed to develop a CPG that covers various aspects of the disease, the contents of the CPG will be outdated and the CPG will not be used widely. If a standard patient is too strictly dealt with and the CPG covers only a small proportion of patients, the CPG also will not be used widely. In both cases, the CPG will not contribute to quality in health care.

3. Design of the Main CPG Framework: Allocation of Subgroups and Medical Interventions

A disease is categorized into subgroups according to subtypes and gravity of the disease. A subgroup should be formed whenever different interventions can be recommended or different prognoses can be expected. For each subgroup, possible medical interventions should be listed. Possibility should be assessed based upon physical and financial accessibility. The main framework of the CPG comprises the subgroups and the optimal medical interventions for each subgroup.

4. Research Questionnaires

Research questionnaires are devised to select the optimal medical intervention for each subgroup. A research questionnaire has four components: patient, intervention, comparison (conventional intervention or placebo), and outcome (PICO).

5. Critical Appraisal or Systemic Evaluation of Papers

To answer the research questionnaires, medical articles are gathered using databases. Medline and Cochrane Library are the most often used databases. Medline is the biggest database in medical fields maintained by the National Library of Medicine in the United States, and contains about 400 million articles from 3500 journals. It contains all kinds of articles. The Cochrane Library is a database specializing in randomized clinical trials (RCTs) and the results of systemic readings. In evidence-based CPG development, RCTs have a key role and the other types of clinical studies have only complementary roles. It is efficient to resort first to the Cochrane Library to gather RCTs and then, if necessary, to use Medline to gather reports of other types of clinical studies.

Papers are ranked as to the power of the evidence based on the study types. Table 1 summarizes the power of the evidence and the degree of recommendation. RCTs are regarded as the most powerful (level I and II), followed by controlled trials with current control groups (level III), controlled trials with historical control groups (level IV), noncontrolled case series, and individual expert's opinions (level V). When evaluating papers, special attention should be paid to outcome indicators; instead of true outcome indicators, surrogates (intermediate indicators) are sometimes used for technical and financial reasons. For example, drugs for hypertension should be evaluated based on the degree to which they lower the occurrence of cerebrovascular events (true outcome) instead of the degree of lowering of blood pressure (surrogate) if the final goal

TABLE 1. Power of evidence and degree of recommendation[a]

Power of evidence		Degree of recommendation	
Level of evidence	Explanation	Degree of recommendation	Explanation
I	Large, randomized clinical trials with clear-cut results (and low risk of error)	A	Supported by at least one, and preferably more than one, level I randomized clinical trial
II	Small, randomized clinical trials with uncertain results (and moderate to high risk of error)	B	Supported by at least one level II randomized clinical trial
III	Nonrandomized, current controls	C	Supported only by level III IV, or V evidence
IV	Nonrandomized, historical controls		
V	No controls, case series only		

[a] Based on Sarkett [1].

of antihypertensive treatment is to prevent cerebrovascular events. A paper using true outcome indicators should be treated as more convincing than one using surrogate indicators, even if they belong to the same rank with regard to the power of the evidence. If a paper reports negative findings, in which the null hypothesis is not denied from the study results, special attention should be paid to whether the number of subjects were sufficient. The RCT has a merit over other types of clinical studies in definitely showing negative results. However, the fact is that many RCTs have an insufficient number of subjects to have a satisfactory power of detection (β equal to or less than 0.20). For example, assuming that intervention A is shown by RCTs using placebos (no intervention) to be effective for treating a disease and a new RCT using interventions A and B reports

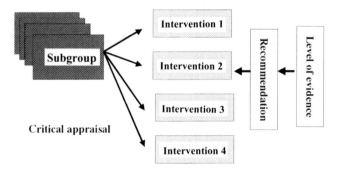

FIG. 1. Structure of clinical practice guidelines. For each subgroup of a disease, interventions currently in practice are evaluated for their effectiveness and efficiency, and only interventions with supporting evidence are recommended

TABLE 2. Economic evaluation of interventions[a]

Name	Cost	Result	Notes
Cost-minimization analysis	Monetary	Same health results are expected	Part of cost-effectiveness analysis when the health results are the same
Cost-effectiveness analysis	Monetary	Health results (life years gained, improvement of pain scores, etc.)	Comparing interventions for different diseases is often difficult, as health results are expressed by different measurements (e.g., life years gained vs. benign prostate hypertrophy urination score improved)
Cost-benefit analysis	Monetary	Monetary Health results are translated into monetary terms	Comparing interventions for different diseases is possible Technical and ethical problems when health results are translated into monetary terms Estimating the absolute monetary balance of introducing the intervention is possible by calculating difference between benefit and cost
Cost-utility analysis	Monetary	Health results are adjusted by utility scores	Quality of life after intervention is taken into consideration Technical, cultural, and ethical problems in estimating quality of life

[a] For details see Drummond et al. [2].

negative results, intervention B will be concluded to be as effective as intervention A for that disease. This may be only because of a lack of a sufficient number of subjects.

Interventions supported by two or more rank I papers are highly recommended (recommendation A). To be recommended, an intervention must have at least one RCT supporting that intervention, which is why the methodology of evidence-based CPG development is highly dependent on RCTs (*RCT absolutism*).

6. Economic Evaluation

Interventions that are evaluated as effective in step 5 need to be evaluated economically. The conditions for economic evaluation are that only interventions shown to be effective are evaluated economically, and economic evaluation is done by comparing two or more interventions. In medicine, physicians sometimes have to contend with diseases related to aging, for which there is no definitive curative treatment. Treating a patient has costs, and the option that minimizes the cost is no treatment. To avoid that pitfall, economic evaluation is performed on the assumption that the patient should be treated and that the most efficient intervention should be selected by comparing possible interventions. Cost-effective, cost-benefit, and cost-utility analyses are representative and the methods used most often. Table 2 describes these three methods.

If only one intervention is effective for a disease, no choice exists medically other than using that intervention. Whether to pay from the public sector is another question relating priority setting among many disease and interventions that public insurance is expected to cover. If one intervention is superior in both health results and cost-efficiency to other interventions, selecting and recommending that intervention is easy. Room for debate exists when one intervention is superior in health results but inferior in cost-efficiency and vice versa. The economic aspect is just one of many values of interventions, and other values should be considered according to the nature of the disease and the interventions. A multidisciplinary process is often used to deal with this complex ethical problem.

7. CPG Development

The CPG is compiled using effective and cost-efficient interventions. Steps 1–6 described here are usually done by several core physicians and a few consulting epidemiologists. A definition of the standard patient for the CPG should be clearly formulated. The flow of patients is expressed by using decision analysis trees, with care providers on each decision analysis tree branch and with explicit criteria to refer the patients from general practitioners to specialists. It is important that the CPG is refined and authorized in a multidisciplinary process that includes representative physicians from specialties responsible for patients with the disease and representatives of governments, payers, and patient associations. Public hearings are sometimes held to gather public comments.

CPGs should be used widely to be effective in clinical settings. Authorization by representatives of related specialties, distribution to physicians in handouts, and websites are sometimes used to promote CPGs among physicians.

8. Medical Intervention Based on CPGs

CPG development is fundamentally a service by specialties to general practitioners to level up medical services. General practitioners treat typical patients based on CPGs and confirm that the expected health results expressed by the CPGs are gained by that treatment. If they use interventions other than those recommended by the CPG, ethically they have a duty to give reasons why they do not follow the CPG. When general practitioners see atypical patients who are not covered by the CPG, they refer these patients to specialists. The proportion of atypical patients who are not covered by the CPG varies by specialty and disease. Specialists treat them with their knowledge and experience, and the CPG is not expected to deal with such infrequent, highly complex cases.

9. Evaluation and Improvement of CPGs

A CPG should be evaluated and improved regularly based on treatment results. Details of evaluation are explained in the following sections.

Characteristics and Limitations of Evidence-Based Medicine

The quality of medical services has been evaluated from three standpoints: structure, process, and outcome [3], and correspondingly, three kinds of approaches to secure quality in medical services are through structure, process, and outcome. Evidence-based medicine is basically a process approach that assumes that a standardized optimal intervention will secure best health results, which should be shown to be effective later. In evaluating CPGs developed by an evidence-based method, special attention must be paid to the following problems.

Structural Problem: The Best Intervention Does Not Always Secure the Best Results

Like other process approaches, evidence-based medicine does not always secure the best results, and the results should be monitored by using appropriate indicators. RCTs are usually conducted with a limited number of subjects in ideal circumstances with skilful physicians and co-medical staffs. The expected effects often cannot be confirmed in clinical settings because of low patient compliance, lack of experience of physicians or co-medical staffs, or both. However, unexpected side effects often occur because RCTs with relatively limited numbers of subjects cannot detect rare side effects. Outcome approaches can and should complement process approaches, including evidence-based medicine.

Technical Problem: Many Clinical Settings Are Not Suitable for RCTs

Although RCT data are almost essential for the development of CPGs by an evidence-based medicine method, many clinical setting are not suitable for RCTs. Some interventions are already being widely used, and some of them are performed on patients at an impaired conscious level, such as hypothermia therapy for traumatic brain damage. These are examples of settings in which RCTs are difficult. The current evidence-based medicine technique is not refined enough and cannot proceed without proper RCT data. It cannot deal with a complex combination of logic. For example, assuming that intervention P is shown to be effective by a large-scale RCT, and that another nonrandomized clinical trial with current controls (level III) reports that both interventions P and Q are equally effective, how can we deal with the intervention Q? It should be recommended as A grade (supported by a RCT) or as C grade (supported by a nonrandomized clinical trial).

Another problem is that evidence-based medicine offers no indication as to the providers who take care of the patients. For example, both internists and urologists take part in treating patients with benign prostate hypertrophy in Japan. No formal curriculum of family medicine exists for general practitioners in Japan. Many internists first work at secondary or tertiary hospitals as specialists, then open their clinics and engage in general internal medicine. Their knowledge and experience is diverse, and predicting their average level of skill in diagnosing and treating patients with urological problems is difficult. With CPGs, the procedure for the evaluation of patient status and the criteria for referring a patient to a specialist should be clearly described. A multidisciplinary process, including representatives of general internal medicine and urology, is important to assure coordination and avoid unnecessary conflicts between the two specialties. A similar problem occurs when CPGs developed abroad are used. Many CPGs are developed in other countries, but importing and using them is difficult because health care systems are different among countries. In addition to scientific components of the CPG, such as lists of papers and results of critical appraisals, and recommended interventions for each subgroup of a disease, we must pay attention to the health insurance system. An intervention covered by health insurance in one country may not be covered in another country.

Framework of Evaluation of CPGs

CPGs should be evaluated on three different levels: the validity in selecting the disease, the validity of the CPG development process, and the impact of CPGs on medicine after their introduction.

Validity in Selecting the Disease

Validity in selecting the disease means that good reasons exist for selecting a disease for CPG development, or that investing resources to develop a CPG for the disease is justified. If a disease has the characteristics described in "selection of disease", it will be prioritized and will be regarded as worth the investment of resources.

There is no single explicit criteria because variations exist in the resources that can be used and in the degree and requests for standardization of health care.

Validity of the CPG Development Process

A CPG should be developed by proper processes, which can be confirmed later. CPGs are expected to have the attributes listed in Table 3. Documentation is important and usually occupies a large part of a CPG. An established CPG is often used as material for a new CPG. If a previously developed CPG has used the same methodology and materials as a new CPG, the new CPG can use the results of the old one. Whether CPGs contain the recommended attributes is fairly easy to see, and many previous studies to evaluate CPGs have used this method.

TABLE 3. Recommended attributes of clinical practice guidelines (CPGs)[a]

Attribute	Explanation
Validity	Methodology by which the CPG is developed is documented, showing data source, means used to evaluated the evidence, results of critical appraisal, and recommended interventions with expected clinical results
Reliability and reproducibility	Reliability and reproducibility are regarded as secured when another set of experts can develop essentially the same CPG if they are given the same evidence and methods; and another physician will select essentially the same intervention if he or she is given the same clinical circumstances
Clinical applicability	A standard patient, to whom the CPG applies, is defined by explicit criteria and is appropriately defined to reflect the majority of the patient population
Clinical flexibility	If several different kinds of values exist in selecting interventions, each recommendation explains the relationship with these values so that a patient's preferences can be respected.
Clarity	CPG is expressed in unambiguous language
Multidisciplinary process	CPG is developed by a multidisciplinary process, including participation of representatives of relevant specialties, governments, payers, and patients
Scheduled review	CPG includes statements of when and by whom to be reviewed and revised
Documentation	Materials and procedures to develop CPGs, participants involved, evidence used, and their strengths must documented in the CPG

[a] The recommended attributes are taken from Field and Lohn [4] but were changed by the author.

Impact of CPGs on Medicine

The final goal of the standardization of health care through evidence-based medicine is to change and improve health care, and the impact of the introduction of CPGs should be evaluated from this point of view. Of the three criteria used to evaluate the quality of health care, CPGs can change two, process and outcome, in two directions: standardization and improvement. They constitute the main part of the quality of health care. CPGs can promote standardization of health care by lessening differences in interventions among physicians (process) and narrowing distributions of indicators, such as prognosis, length of stay, and costs (outcome). They can also improve absolute values reflecting the outcome of interventions, such as survival rate, number of unexpected admissions, length of stay, and costs (Table 4).

The evaluation of CPGs from this standpoint so far is limited. Most studies reporting improved quality of health care are limited to a few diseases and have to use historical controls. An appropriate study design to evaluate the impact of introducing CPGs should be developed. Establishing a patient registration system to evaluate the impact of CPGs is essential. Evidence-based medicine is

TABLE 4. Impact of clinical practice guidelines on medicine

Standpoint	Process		Outcome
Emphasis	Promotion of standardization (narrowing of distribution)		Improvement of absolute value
Examples	Lessening differences of intervention among physicians	Narrowing of distribution in indicators, such as prognosis, length of stay, and health care costs	Improvement of absolute value in indicators, such as prognosis, length of stay, and health care costs
	Increase in compliance with standardized interventions (CPGs, clinical paths)		

powerful and seems easy to learn, but it is a process approach, and the impact of the process approach should be measured by a highly useful indicator: the outcome.

References

1. Sackett DL (1989) Rules of evidence and clinical recommendations on the use of antithrombotic agents. Chest 95(2) Suppl: 2S–4S
2. Drummond MF, O'Brien B, Stoddart GL, Torrance GW (1997) Methods for the economic evaluation of healthcare programmes, 2nd edn. Oxford University Press, Oxford
3. Donabedian A (1966) Evaluating the quality of medical care. Milbank Mem Fund Q 44(3) Suppl: 166–206
4. Field MJ, Lohr KN (eds) (1992) CPGs for clinical practice. National Academy Press, Washington, DC

Fundamentals and Role of Clinical Pathway in Clinical Guidelines: Application of a Clinical Pathway for Transurethral Resection of the Prostate

Yoshihiro Nagata[1] and Shuhei Iida[2]

Summary. A clinical pathway for transurethral resection of the prostate was developed at Nerima General Hospital in 1999 in response to an excessive length of hospitalization and an increase in the overall hospital costs in comparison to one year previously for patients undergoing transurethral resection of the prostate. A multidisciplinary team was formed to develop, implement, and monitor the use of a clinical pathway for patients undergoing transurethral resection of the prostate for benign prostatic hypertrophy. Through such multidisciplinary collaboration, the length of hospitalization and hospital costs were successfully reduced, while the quality care indicators were all maintained. This chapter describes the development of this clinical pathway and also demonstrates the outcomes after implementation.

Key Words. Clinical pathway, Transurethral resection of prostate, Length of hospitalization, Hospital charge

Introduction

The concept of developing clinical pathways originated in the construction and engineering fields, where it proved a valuable tool for managing large, complex projects [1]. Clinical pathways, which have been reported as a tool to monitor health care outcomes and have emerged as a successful strategy for improving the quality and effectiveness of health care, were first introduced in the 1970s and gained prominence in the 1980s at the New England Medical Center [2].

Another pioneer in nursing care management was Hillcrest Medical Center, where the purpose of the clinical pathway was to guide patient care. Others have reported the use of this methodology for coronary bypass patients, orthopedic care, neonatal intensive care, trauma, emergency care, treatment of neurological

[1]Department of Urology, [2]Department of Surgery, Nerima General Hospital, 2-24-1 Asahigaoka, Nerima-ku, Tokyo 176-8530, Japan

---

1. Clinical pathways
2. Critical pathways
3. Case maps
4. Anticipated recovery plans
5. Multidisciplinary care plans

FIG. 1. Common names for clinical pathways

patients, and urological disease [3–14]. Clinical pathways have also been called critical pathways, care maps, anticipated recovery plans, and multidisciplinary plans (Fig. 1).

Multiple factors have contributed to the emergence of clinical pathways in various health care settings, including changes in hospital reimbursement procedures, increased emphasis on multidisciplinary interactions, rising malpractice costs, and mounting evidence of wide variations in clinical practice.

Clinical pathways are typically developed for high-volume, high-cost, high-risk, and problem-prone patient populations in the medical field. They are also a set of expectations for the major components of care that a patient should receive to manage a specific medical or surgical diagnosis. Clinical pathways outline the nursing care plans, laboratory tests, medications, and therapies that are essential to produce the desired outcome and seek to eliminate any waste associated with medical procedures at various medical institutions. They also incorporate the care requirement of all the clinical disciplines involved in a patient's care.

The substantial excessive costs from nonessential laboratory tests, extended hospitalization, unnecessary medications, inadequate pain control, and other factors can all be decreased by standardizing specific nursing and medication protocols and by educating and motivating patients to follow a carefully planned program for both preoperative and postoperative management. In short, clinical pathways define the necessary components of medical care that are involved in the process of care, thus resulting in a shorter hospitalization and decreased hospital costs [15–17]. As a result of using appropriate clinical pathways, the patients, family, and hospital staff can all benefit. Hart and Musfeldt assert that the consistency afforded by the use of clinical pathways increases the efficiency of time, decreases cost, and effectively integrates multiple medical services [18] (Fig. 2).

Based on these theories of clinical pathways, a clinical pathway for transurethral resection of the prostate was developed at the Department of Urology, Nerima General Hospital, to reduce the length of hospitalization and decrease hospital costs.

Clinical Pathway Development Process

The implementation of clinical pathways at both the Department of Urology and the urological ward of Nerima General Hospital was initiated in 1999. The goals of a clinical pathway are to improve the effective management and

1. Improvement in patient outcome
2. Improved quality and continuity of care
3. Improvement in multidisciplinary communication and collaboration
4. Identification of organizational system problems
5. Coordination of necessary services and reduced duplication
6. Prioritization of care activities
7. Decreased hospitalization and lower costs

FIG. 2. Potential benefits of clinical pathways

1. Select clinical pathway
2. Identify team facilitator to conduct groundwork
3. Collect information from:
   a) other institutions' available path examples
   b) length of hospitalization
   c) chart review
   d) literature review
   e) other diagnosis-related documents, such as care plans, protocols, or guidelines
4. Collect information on:
   a) length of hospitalization
   b) hospital costs
   c) complications
   d) recommended practice patterns
   e) current practice patterns
   f) miscellaneous
5. Compile all information and develop a rough outline of the path. An outline will offer the team a starting point

FIG. 3. Phase I: Groundwork

care involved in the transurethral resection of the prostate associated with high costs, excessive hospitalization, and the use of unnecessary medications, as compared with the year before the initiation of clinical pathway. Attending urologists and several nursing specialists from the urological ward staff were selected to develop a clinical pathway for our population of patients with benign prostatic hypertrophy. The clinical pathway development process was conducted as follows.

Phase I: Groundwork

The development of a clinical pathway typically proceeds in five phases: groundwork, team selection, team meetings, approval, and education and implementation. During the groundwork phase, data are collected to evaluate the length of hospitalization, hospital costs, complications, and quality issues (Fig. 3). As a result of such data analysis, our institution's length of hospitalization was found to be 17.15 days before the use of a clinical pathway for transurethral resection of the prostate. Although postoperative management was carefully carried out, variations in practice, related to injection of the antibiotics, fluid administration, diet progression, and catheter removal, all contributed to an unnecessarily long hospitalization. As a result, there was no clinical protocol for the patient's postoperative course. To establish a clinical pathway for transurethral resection of the prostate, the attending urologist and associate team members used documented principles of surgical recovery to draft a clinical pathway according to the standard format for clinical pathways used at our institution. This draft pathway provided the basis for team discussions and further development in phase II.

Phase II: Team Selection

The groundwork was followed by the selection of members of a multidisciplinary team who were responsible for the clinical pathway as well as for reviewing, developing, and implementing a variation in the analysis data, formulating plans of action, performing ongoing critiques, and revising the clinical pathway when necessary. The clinical pathway team for transurethral resection of the prostate at our institution included attending urologists, nursing specialists for urological care and management, pharmacists, dieticians, laboratory technicians, and radiology technicians (Fig. 4).

Phase III: Team Meetings

Team meetings provided an opportunity to discuss patient care and evaluate the draft clinical pathway. The draft should be carefully reviewed and analyzed before the first meeting. Several meetings should be held to overcome problems and fine-tune the clinical pathway. The first meeting should determine each member's goals for the clinical pathway and discuss the discharge outcome for the patients. A second meeting should develop a draft of the clinical pathway based on the feedback from discussion of all problems, and the draft should be revised accordingly. A third meeting should review the feedback and make appropriate revisions. In our case, however, we recognized that time constraints prevented the attendance of useful hospital members, such as physicians for diabetes and medical office staff members. We therefore met individually with such members to establish a thorough clinical pathway for transurethral resection of the prostate and allow all members to clearly express their ideas. Feedback was delivered to our team, and pathway revisions were made accordingly.

---

1. Determine process for team selection
2. The steering committee can select the members and/or facilitator
3. Contact team members and outline project
4. Hold several meetings

FIG. 4. Phase II: Team selection

1. The clinical pathway should be approved by urologists whose patients will be placed on the pathway. Direct approval can be obtained from each urologist, or approval may be obtained from an appropriate medical committee
2. The clinical pathway should be approved by any necessary institutional committees

Fig. 5. Phase IV: Approval of clinical pathway

1. Plan for printing and distributing pathways
2. Determine what contents need to be addressed to education
3. Develop method for education, as follows:
   a) demonstrations of clinical pathway implementation
   b) case studies to verify understanding
   c) explanations using posters and flowchart
4. Clearly announce implementation date and education plans to team members and appropriate physicians
5. Implement the clinical pathway

Fig. 6. Phase VI: Education and implementation

Phase IV: Approval of the Clinical Pathway

Once a working version of the clinical pathway was developed, formal input and approval were solicited from all urologists at our institution who were involved in the care of patients with benign prostate hypertrophy. Opportunities were provided for each urologist to suggest modifications to the clinical pathway (Fig. 5).

Phase V: Education and Implementation

After the urologists' approval of the clinical pathway had been received, a plan was designed for education and implementation of the new pathway. Education began with the nursing staffs of the urological ward under the direction of the urologists. For example, a demonstration of the clinical pathway implementation and explanations using posters and flowcharts of the clinical pathway process were used to teach staff how to implement the pathway in daily practice. The education was facilitated by the placement of most patients with benign prostatic hypertrophy in the urological ward (Figs. 6, 7).

Method, Outcomes, and Role of Clinical Pathway for Transurethral Resection of Prostate at Nerima General Hospital

The end product of the development process was a clinical pathway for transurethral resection of the prostate, and it has resulted in a shorter hospitalization and decreased hospital costs. Our clinical pathway is divided into 14 days,

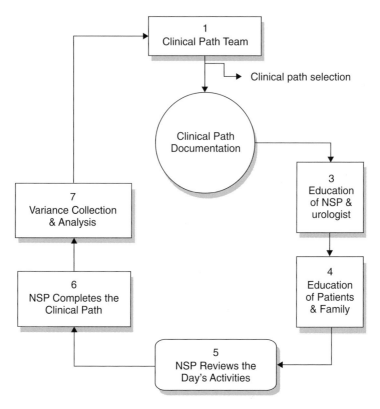

FIG. 7. Transurethral prostatectomy clinical path implementation flowchart. *NSP*, nurse specialist

and appropriate items in the clinical pathway are listed in the following eight categories: treatment; medications; observation, including a check of vital signs; laboratory tests, such as complete blood count and blood chemistry; activity; nutrition; education; and variance (Fig. 8).

Based on the clinical pathway process, we treated patients with benign prostate hypertrophy. At hospitalization, nurse specialists in the urological ward educated the patient and his family about the pre- and postoperation process. All preoperative tests were ordered in the outpatient department and were performed about 20 days before admission to the hospital. Data from the preoperative tests were collected before the day of operation. The nurse specialists also reviewed the patients' daily activity and recorded it daily on the clinical pathway form. The operating room was prepared for the patient according to the schedule of the urologists. The method of anesthesia was determined by an anesthesiologist prior to the operation. Most patients received epidural block anesthesia. Intravenous fluid was administered at about 9:00 A.M. on the day of operation. Blood transfusion was given during the operation if a large amount of bleeding was noticed.

Nerima General Hospital
Departmet of Urology
Title: TUR-P

Pt's name: _____
Attending Dr: _____

	Before admission	Admission	Operation	POD 1	POD 2	POD 3	POD 4
Treatment		Nursing preparation	• ECG monitor if necessary • O₂ inspiration if necessary • Transfusion if necessary • Bladder irrigation • On 3-way Foley	D/C ———→ D/C ———→ ————→ ————→ ————→			Removed Foley
Medications		Fleet enema Laxative P.O.	• Antibiotics (intravenous administration) • Analgesic (IM or suppository if needed)		←—— ←——		Antibiotics (Oral)
Observation (vital signs)			q0.5h × 2 q1h × 2 q2h × 2 then q4–6h	q4–6h		D/C	
Tests	Chest X-P ECG CBC, blood chemistry HB-Ags, HCV, Wa U/A		CBC, BUN, Na, K, Cl (sugar)	CBC Blood chemistry			CBC, blood chemistry, U/A
Activity		Ambulate	Bed rest	Ambulate	D/C		Take shower
Nutrition		NPO since 9:00 pm	N.P.O.	Diet as tolerated	D/C		
Education		Orientation pre/postop teaching	D/C				
				Continue	Continue		
Variance							

Fig. 8. Clinical path form for transurethral resection of the prostate (original form in Japanese). NPO, nothing orally; D/C, discontinue; CBC, complete blood count; U/A, urinalysis; POD, postoperative day; BUN, blood urea nitrogen

29

When there was any deviation between the expected and actual treatment plan, the nurse specialist in the urological ward identified it and recorded it on the clinical pathway form. After the patient was discharged from the hospital, a nurse specialist in the urological ward completed the clinical pathway documentation and sent it to the clinical pathway team for analysis. Biweekly meetings were held to discuss the variance date and methods to resolve problems. Finally, the clinical pathway team members reported the results to the urologists as a reference for future updating of the clinical pathway. Variance data and the results of various analyses were stored at the office of the clinical pathway members.

From January to December 2000, 72 consecutive patients with benign prostatic hypertrophy were treated by urologists according to the above clinical pathway for transurethral resection of the prostate. The results after clinical pathway implementation were compared to those of 67 consecutive patients treated by urologists from January to December 1997 before use of the clinical pathway.

Student's t-test was used to evaluate the statistical significance of differences before and after implementation of the clinical pathway. The 67 patients treated before the clinical pathway was implemented ranged from 69 to 90 years of age (average, 76.2 years), and the 72 patients treated after use of the clinical pathway ranged from 61 to 87 years of age (average, 74.2). There was no significant difference in the age between the two groups. The length of hospitalization at our institution was 17.15 days before use of the clinical pathway for transurethral resection of the prostate and 14.13 days after the use of the clinical pathway, a statistically significant 17.6 % decrease in the length of hospitalization ($P < 0.02$). The main reason for the decrease in length of hospitalization was considered the effective management of catheter removal after transurethral resection of the prostate and the optimal starting time of oral antibiotic administration instead of intravenous antibiotic administration. In our study, the implementation of the clinical pathway also reduced the number of unnecessary medical procedures. We found that the length of hospitalization, admission fee, and laboratory expenditures decreased after the implementation of the clinical pathway (Table 1).

Similar to the findings of previous studies, our results demonstrate that the

TABLE 1. Mean length of hospital stay and admission charges for patients undergoing transurethral resection of prostate

Category	Before implementation	After implementation	P value
LOS (days)	17.15	14.13	0.002
Charges (Japanese yen)			
Admission fee	287 220	238 073	0.029
Laboratory	26 267	22 547	0.076
Radiology	18 977	11 738	0.010
Oral administration	11 361	13 806	0.175
Intravenous administration	31 020	30 561	0.883

LOS, length of hospital stay.

implementation of a clinical pathway could effectively control medical care expenditures [19–22]. The impact of reducing the length of hospitalization and medical care expenditures on the quality of care remains the greatest concern. Schriefer reported lower readmission and mortality rates, as well as reduced length of hospitalization and medical expenditures, after the implementation of a clinical pathway for coronary artery bypass grafts [23]. A decrease in the number of urinary tract infections and a reduced rate of aspiration pneumonia, as well as improved quality of care, were also noted after the implementation of a clinical pathway for nonhemorrhagic stroke.

We conclude that use of the urologists involved in the clinical pathway for transurethral resection of the prostate can improve health care outcome by reducing the length of hospitalization and associated costs, while also improving the quality of care. We believe that as a greater number of clinical pathways are implemented, both hospital efficiency and quality of care can be improved.

References

1. Turley K, Tyndall M, Roge C, Cooper M, Turley K, Applebaum M, Tarnoff H (1994) Critical pathway methodology: effectiveness in congenital heart surg. Ann Thorac Surg 58:57–65
2. Zander K (1988) Managed care within acute care setting: design and implementation via nursing case management. Health Care Superv 6(2):27–43
3. Flickinger JE, Trusler L, Brock JW (1997) Clinical care pathway for the management of ureteroneocystostomy in the pediatric urology population. J Urol 158:1221–1225
4. Heacock A, Brobst RA (1994) A multidisciplinary approach to critical path development: a valuable CQI tool. J Nurs Care Qual 8:38–47
5. Barnes RV, Lawton L, Briggs D (1994) Clinical benchmarking improves clinical paths: experience with coronary artery bypass grafting. Jt Comm J Qual Improv 20:267–276
6. Shikiar MS, Warner P (1994) Selecting financial indices to measure critical path outcomes. Nurs Manage 25:58–60
7. Zander K (1990) Managed care and nursing case management. Aspen Publications
8. McKenzie CB, Torkelson NG, Holt MA (1995) Care and cost. Nurs Manage 20:30–34
9. Strong AG, Sneed NV (1991) Clinical evaluation of a critical path for coronary artery bypass surgery patients. Prog Cardiovasc Nurs 6:29–35
10. Metcalf EM (1991) The orthopedic critical path. Orthop Nurs 10:25–31
11. Latini EE, Foote W (1992) Obtaining consistent quality patient care for the trauma patient by using a critical pathway. Crit Care Nurs Q 15:51–55
12. Neidig JR, Megel ME, Koehler KM (1992) The critical path: an evaluation of the application of nursing care management in the NICU. Neonatal Netw 11:45–52
13. Nelson MS (1993) Critical pathway in the emergency department. J Emerg Nurse 19:110–114
14. Richards JS, Sonda LP, Gaucher E, Kocan MJ, Ross D (1993) Applying critical pathways to neurosurgery patients at the University of Michigan Medical Center. Qual Lett Health Lead 5:8–10
15. Holtzman J, Bjerke T, Kane R (1998) The effects of clinical pathways for renal transplantation on patient outcomes and length of stay. Med Care 36:826–834

16. Keetch DW, Buback D (1998) A clinical-care pathway for decreasing hospital stay after radical prostatectomy. Br J Urol 81:398–402
17. Chang PL, Wang TM, Huang ST, Hsieh ML, Tsui KH (1999) Effect of implementation of 18 clinical pathways on costs and quality of care among patients undergoing urological surgery. J Urol 161:1858–1862
18. Hart R, Musfeldt C (1992) MD-directed critical pathways: it's time. Hospitals 63: 56
19. Lindstrom CC, Laird J, Socia J (1995) High quality and lower cost. They can coexist. Semin Nurse Manage 3:133–136
20. Simundson S, Lavoie D (1994) Clinical paths at Rhode Island Hospital: tool for outcome management. American Hospital Publishing, Chicago, pp 81–97
21. Spath PL (1995) Critical paths: maximizing patient care coordination. Today OR Nurse 17:13–20
22. Chang PL, Huang ST, Hsieh ML, Wang TM, Chen JI, Kuo HH, Chuang YC, Chang CH (1997) Use of the transurethral prostatectomy clinical path to monitor health outcomes. J Urol 157:177–183
23. Schriefer J (1994) The synergy of pathways and algorithms: two tools work better than one. Jt Comm J Qual Improv 20:485–499

Technical Evaluation and Its Ethics for New Interventional Treatment

RALPH V. CLAYMAN[1] and THOMAS H. GALLAGHER[2]

Summary. Technical innovation presents a major ethical challenge for the practicing physician. Conflicts of interest, both academic and financial, need to be identified and addressed on the institutional, professional, and patient level. On the institutional and professional level, regulations regarding the investigation of new devices and disclosure of physician–industrial relationships can help insure physician propriety. On the patient level, there is general agreement that patients should be informed of physician–industrial relationships. However, the best strategy for disclosing such conflicts of interest to patients is unclear. When evaluating his or her relationships with industry, the best interests of the patient should always guide the physician. In years to come, the ethics for new interventional treatment will probably involve disclosing potential conflicts of interest to patients, colleagues, and institutions to a greater degree than in years past.

Key Words. Disclosure, Conflict of interest, Ethics, Technical innovation

Introduction

The development and dissemination of innovative medical technologies has produced enormous benefits for patients and for society at large. Physicians involved with the development and testing of new technologies face a variety of competing pressures. The successful dissemination of a new technology can bring academic and financial rewards to the physician. However, patients may be harmed if they are subjected to technologies that prove to be ineffective. Even in the absence of harm to patients, some commentators worry that overly strong financial relationships between physicians and industry could damage patients' trust in their physicians and in the medical profession. In this chapter we discuss this

[1] Department of Urology, University of California (Irvine), 101 The City Drive, Building 55, Room 304, Route 81, Orange, CA 92868, USA
[2] Division of General Medical Sciences, Washington University School of Medicine, 660 S. Euclid Avenue, St. Louis, MO 63110, USA

conflict and its control in general terms and then proceed to further examine the impact of these conflicts as they relate to physicians' relationships with their patients, their colleagues, and their institutions.

Conflicts of Interest

The primary concern about relationships between physicians and industry is the potential for conflicts of interest [1,2]. These conflicts are typically generated by financial ties between physicians and industry. Such ties may be as seemingly innocuous as support to attend a meeting or on a larger scale: laboratory support, speaker's board, consulting fees, royalties, and/or stock options or ownership. Financial ties between physicians and industry are increasingly common. In one study, nearly 10% of faculty reported personal financial ties with the sponsors of their research [3]. The potential for financial arrangements to unduly influence physicians' decisions has been a source of concern for the professional and lay public for many years. In his 1913 play "The Doctor's Dilemma: A Tragedy," George Bernard Shaw describes the problem of conflicts of interest in medicine:

As to the honor and conscience of doctors, they have as much as any other class of men, no more and no less. And what other men dare pretend to be impartial where they have a strong pecuniary interest on one side? Nobody supposes that doctors are less virtuous than judges; but a judge whose salary and reputation depended on whether the verdict was for plaintiff or defendant, prosecutor or prisoner, would be as little trusted as a general in the pay of the enemy. To offer me a doctor as my judge, and then weight his decision with a bribe of a large sum of money ... is to go wildly beyond the ascertained strain which human nature will bear. [4]

Conflicts of interest in medicine could have a variety of alarming outcomes [5,6]. Most worrisome would be if the conflict impaired the physician's judgment and resulted in the proffering of a therapy that is of no benefit or even harmful to the patient. On occasion this bias in a physician's judgment can be the result of a conscious decision to place his or her financial interests ahead of the needs of the patient. More commonly, however, financial ties influence physicians' behavior subconsciously, distorting the decisions of well-meaning and conscientious physicians. In addition, even absent evidence that conflicts of interest are actually affecting physicians' decisions, some financial arrangements may create the appearance of a conflict of interest, undermining trust in the medical profession. In this situation, the fact and the perception of a conflict of interest indistinguishably merge until the problem is one of "perception is reality." How can physicians respond to these potential conflicts of interest in their relationships with industry?

Ethics of Technical Responsibility

The ethics of technical responsibility spring from the relationship of physicians to their patients, professional colleagues, and institutions. At each level there are a different set of concerns that need to be addressed when the physician accepts a relationship with industry. From the patient standpoint, the physician involved in technical evaluation has several concerns. Specifically, the physician's interest in applying the new technology must be counterbalanced by two other important aspects: issues of technology application, and disclosure of potential conflicts of interest. At a professional level, the physician involved in technical development must be concerned about the accurate and clear reporting of device-related data and the issue of full disclosure to his or her colleagues. Lastly, at the institutional level, the physician needs to have insured that prior to initiating a study of the proposed product, all institutional requirements have been met. These include approval of the project by the Investigational Review Board, maintenance of study books and signed informed consents, and disclosure of any agreements or contracts between the physician and the company producing the product.

The patient–physician relationship with regard to device development revolves around two central factors: issues of technology application, and disclosure of conflicts of interest. The unique nature of the doctor–patient relationship requires that physicians first and foremost do what is in the patient's best interest. Therefore, with regard to the *application* of a new technology, physicians must first ensure that the device in question will benefit patients. Although this seems simplistic and obvious, there are unfortunately numerous instances in our surgical history where surgeons have ignored this principle in pursuit of new technology; in the long run, the technology has failed and patients have suffered.

The American College of Surgeons has recently produced a statement regarding application of new technology to patient care. In this statement, four questions need to be answered prior to use of the new technology: 1) "Has the new technology been adequately tested for safety and efficacy?", 2) "Is the new technology at least as safe and effective as existing, proven techniques?", 3) "Is the individual proposing to perform the new procedure fully qualified to do so?", and 4) "Is the new technology cost-effective?" [7]. Prior to the release of any product, single-center or preferably multicenter trials with the device are completed and the results are published. It is the responsibility of each physician to carefully review these papers to determine the adequacy of the trial and the safety as well as the efficacy of the given device; only when these aspects have been definitively addressed and answered in the affirmative is it reasonable for the prudent physician to proceed to the next step of learning how to use the device. Training may be as simple as an in-service with the company representative (e.g., a new guidewire) or as complex as attending a hands-on course followed by a clinical mentor/proctor experience (e.g., vascular bypass stents).

Attention to the first three items of the American College of Surgeons statement is in the interest of patient safety and efficacy; the last item is one of financial benefit and is more difficult to assess. Cost-effectiveness is a commonly used term in today's health-care-conscious environment, yet of all of the previously discussed factors, it is the most difficult to define, because the costs of a product are myriad and often difficult to discern. As such, in most cases, a device is adopted for clinical use based on a "Yes" answer to the first three questions; the concern over cost-effectiveness is often not answered until the device has been used extensively in clinical practice.

Once the physician has decided that the device is ready for human use, the physician must share whatever information the patient needs to make an informed choice about whether to proceed with the recommended device, the process known as informed consent. Although physicians are accustomed to sharing clinical information with patients as part of informed consent, they should also *disclose* to patients the relationship of the physician to the company producing the product for which a given treatment is recommended. Disclosure is an important and inseparable part of the informed consent process. The physician, by law, is required to reveal to the patient all known alternatives of therapy, with their attendant benefits and risks; by the same token, the physician must also reveal to the patient any other interests that could possibly affect his or her recommendation. Such disclosure is presumed to have two beneficial effects. First, being aware of the relationship between the physician and the device manufacturer may help patients make more informed choices about whether to proceed with the recommended therapy. In addition, the need to disclose potential conflicts of interest may have a deterrent effect, encouraging physicians to avoid relationships with industry they would be uncomfortable explaining to patients. Therefore, full disclosure of any potential conflicts of interest with regard to a given therapy is part and parcel of the informed consent process.

Conflicts of interest are not necessarily purely financial. Physicians often face incentives to treat that are scientific as well as financial. The two are often inextricably mixed, specifically when a device is in the trial stage. Scientifically, the physician is involved in an effort to determine the worth of a new therapy. In order to do this, patients need to be recruited to participate in either a longitudinal study of safety and efficacy or a prospective, randomized endeavor to determine the worthiness of a given device compared with standard therapy. These studies are the source of subsequent publications and presentations, thereby contributing to an individual's academic reputation. The spin-off results in academic promotion, further scientific studies, patient referrals, and attraction of postgraduate students at the resident and fellow level. From a financial standpoint, there are many concerning aspects operating at both a tangible and subconscious level. The investigating physician often receives the device free of charge to use; this in and of itself provides the physician with a financial edge as well as a potential marketing tool, for providing his or her patients with the "latest and greatest" therapy for a disease before it is available to the general medical community. In addition, the investigating physician may be receiving a stipend for each patient recruited into the study or for each patient undergoing therapy with the device; the compensation for this activity funds the clinical investigation and may help fund other laboratory activities [8,9]. Future royalty agreements, as well as the worth of stock options, may be dependent upon the success of the device.

Although there is general agreement that potential conflicts of interest should be disclosed to patients, the best strategy for accomplishing such disclosure has not been codified. Even as a part of informed consent for a new device or therapy, the document presented to the patient often contains no information regarding any relationship between the physician and the company producing the device or drug. Certainly, disclosure in the routine office setting is similarly nonexistent. We have yet to see a document listing an individual physician's company financial relations that has been prepared for distribution to patients; similarly, we have not encountered a physician who has informed us that this is a routine part of his or her initial contact with a patient. But times are changing, and a physician's worthiness and integrity are no longer assumed by an educated and anxious patient population; disclosure of this nature could well go a long way to restoring patient trust.

The concern over conflicts of interest is significant and growing within the health care community. However, even with a full and careful disclosure of the relevant conflicts, the physician may still have a bias in favor of the device-related treatment, leaving the patient in an undecided state. Indeed, it has been suggested that physicians with financial interests in a given product or therapy consider removing themselves from the patient decision-making process entirely, by recommending that the patient seek a second opinion from a qualified physician who has no financial interest in or other ties to the proposed therapy [10].

At a professional level, the physician involved in new device testing or implementation has two responsibilities to the physician community: scientific accuracy and financial disclosure. With regard to scientific accuracy, the conduct and reporting of the study must not be encumbered by the sponsoring company. To this end, the physician must be free to design a proper scientific study to assess all reasonable aspects of a device with regard to its safety and efficacy. A poorly done or compromised study is of no value to the scientific or health care community; indeed, in urology there are several examples with regard to therapy of benign prostatic hypertrophy in which ill-conceived laboratory studies have led to clinical studies of a similar nature, with the resultant widespread use of a device; in time, the lack of efficacy of the device became all too apparent to practitioners, and it was withdrawn from the market. It is the responsibility of the physician to preclude this scenario. Accurate data collection and the institution of studies that can objectively evaluate a technology are essential to the protection of the public and the individual maintenance of physician integrity. The data accumulated should be reviewed and assessed by an independent party; any discrepancies between an independent reviewer's assessment of the data and that of the primary paid investigator must be resolved prior to its publication or presentation. Along these same lines, it is important that no study should ever become the sole property of the sponsoring industry; the investigating physician must be free to report his or her findings at meetings and in the scientific press. Although the sponsoring company certainly may request the right to read, review, and comment on findings prior to their formal presentation, and even may request a brief delay in their presentation to the public, their eventual reporting should not be suppressed. These arrangements between physician and sponsoring industry must be made clear prior to initiation of any research relationship.

Financial disclosure to colleagues, up front and in advance of presenting data, is the glue of professional relationships, which in turn are based on trust and integrity. In the long run, there are no secrets. It is incumbent upon the investigator to inform his or her colleagues of any and all financial relationships he or she may have to a given product. Royalties, speaker honoraria, stock ownership, stock options, research support, or membership on a company's board can be succinctly disclosed at the beginning of any presentation or accompanying any manuscript. Indeed, such disclosure is now required by all CME-accredited courses. It is truly a poor reflection on the medical profession that an action so obvious and vital to honest communication with one's colleagues has needed to be removed from the realm of moral character and made into a rule in order to enforce proper disclosure. On a professional level, there is no more precious possession that any physician has than integrity; it is a gift bestowed by public and professional trust; by the same token, once compromised, no amount of money or sacrifice can achieve its return.

At the university level, the academic and financial aspects of physician–industry interaction are overseen by several committees. At all universities, an Investigational Review Board is the scientific watchdog of the academic health care community. Each clinical study is carefully reviewed to determine proper study design, accurate and understandable informed consent, and satisfaction of all national regulatory requirements [e.g., Investigation Device Exemption (IDE) number by the Federal Drug Administration in the United States]. In addition, in certain circumstances, the protocol may be reviewed by the university's Ethics Committee. From a financial standpoint, most universities have now created a Disclosure Committee to which each member of the university is required to submit an annual report of any and all financial arrangements with industry [11–13]. Indeed, in many centers, no contract with industry can be signed by an individual until it has been reviewed by the university's legal staff and approved. The determination of significant conflicts of interest by this committee may result in alteration of a scientific endeavor such that independent safeguards (i.e., reviewers with no financial incentive) are included in the protocol.

The university or hospital can deal with disclosed conflicts of interest in one of three ways: banning, regulation, or laissez-faire. In the first example, the university or credentialing hospital may decide that a particular class of conflicts of interest is too worrisome. For instance, the university or hospital may forbid its physicians to own stock in any medical device company or prevent them from serving as a paid consultant for any company. Alternatively, a more moderate stance may be adopted: regulation. However, to do this, the university or hospital needs to establish a committee on physician–industry relationships and require all physicians to complete a disclosure form for annual review. The committee can then decide the inherent risk in each conflict of interest and make recommendations as to which relationships need to be altered or ended. For instance, while stock options may be permissible, they may be limited to a certain dollar amount or laboratory support in excess of a particular level would result in the need for independent review of the resulting data prior to publication. In the last case, the university or hospital may elect to have no active participation in physician–industry liasons. In this example, the university or hospital would either adopt a "don't ask, don't tell" policy or request that an annual disclosure statement be completed and kept on file.

Summary

In the final analysis, we come back to Shaw. The recognition of human frailty in the face of financial incentives is what has led the legal profession to create rules and regulations on appropriate and inappropriate interactions. These laws are designed to prevent judges or other officials from participating in a case in which they have a personal interest, either perceived or real; by this action the legal profession seeks to preserve and promote the public's faith in the integrity of the judicial system. How can the medical profession presume to be any less vulnerable? Although no physician should have to excuse himself or herself from providing a patient with care, proper disclosure and, if need be, recommending a second opinion, is certainly within the realm of reason. Through reaffirmation of the primacy of patient care and appropriate, complete disclosure, it is certainly possible for us all, as a profession, to remedy "The Doctor's Dilemma" and transform it from "Tragedy" to "Triumph."

References

1. Rodwin MM (1993) Medicine, money, and morals (Physicians' conflicts of interest). Oxford University Press, New York
2. Lo B (2000) Resolving ethical dilemmas: a guide for clinicians. Lippincott Williams and Wilkins, New York
3. Boyd EA, Bero LA (2000) Assessing faculty financial relationships with industry. JAMA 284:2209–2214
4. Shaw GB (1965) The doctor's dilemma: a tragedy. Penguin Books, Baltimore, pp 8–9
5. Korn D (2000) Conflicts of interest in biomedical research. JAMA 284:2233–2236
6. Martin JB, Kasper DL (2000) In whose best interest? Breaching the academic industrial wall. N Engl J Med 343:1646–1649
7. Statement from the American College of Surgeons (1995) Bull Am Coll Surgeons. 80(9):46–47
8. Farrow GA (1989) Ethics of funding clinical investigation. Can J Surg 32:320
9. DeAngelis CD (2000) Conflict of interest and the public trust. JAMA 284:2237–2238
10. Rowdin MA (1989) Sounding board: physicians' conflicts of interest. N Engl J Med 321:1405–1408
11. McCrary SV, Anderson CB, Jakovlievic J, Khan T, McCullough LB, Wnay NP, Brody BA (2000) A national survey of policies on disclosure of conflicts of interest in biomedical research. N Engl J Med 343:1621–1626
12. Cho MK, Shohara R, Schissel A, Rennie D (2000) Policies on faculty conflicts of interest at US universities. JAMA 284:2203–2208
13. Lo B, Wolf LE, Berkely A (2000) Conflict-of-interest policies for investigators in clinical trials. N Engl J Med 343:1616–1620

Issues in Clinical Studies for Development of Medical Devices in Japan

Nobuhiko Hata and Takeyoshi Dohi

Summary. We summarize the issues on clinical studies for medical device development unique to Japan. The administrative law to approve medical devices, the Pharmaceutical Affairs Law, its administrative agency, the Ministry for Health, Labor, and Welfare (MHLW), and other supporting regulatory institutions are also introduced. We also describe government initiatives to promote the development of medical devices. Standards on the Implementation of Clinical Trials on Drugs, or New GCO by the MHLW, the Translational Research Center of the Ministry of Education, Culture, Sports, Science, and Technology, and two projects by the Ministry of Economy, Trade, and Industry. The development of medical devices is facilitated by bringing together multidisciplinary researchers and clinicians. Effort is needed to fill the gap between governing agencies and to make clinical trial regulation visible not only to industry but also to researchers and clinicians.

Key Words. Clinical study, Medical device, Collaborative research, Government initiative

Introduction

Clinical progress depends on advances in science and technology, such as computer science, nano-technology, opto-electronics, and mechatronics. For example, surgical robots achieve micro- to millimeter-scale surgical maneuvering under the computerized control of advanced medical imaging. As advanced medical devices emerge and commercial products are developed, government regulations have to cope with their rapid change. However, government regulations requiring that the device be carefully examined in clinical applications with large numbers of subjects are contradictory to the rapid improvement of technology outside of

Department of Mechano-Informatics, University of Tokyo, Graduate School of Information Science and Technology, 7-3-1 Hongo, Bunkyo-ku, Tokyo 113-8656, Japan medicine, thus harming the possibility of bringing the best possible medical treatment to patients. Therefore, administrative procedures for the regulatory approval of medical devices and clinical studies should be carefully designed and implemented. A unique issue in Japan is that the regulatory process is lengthy, thus limiting the introduction of foreign medical products into the Japanese market [1].

This chapter summarizes the unique issues concerning clinical studies for the development of medical devices in Japan. We also report the Japanese government's effort to improve clinical studies for applications of medical devices.

Standards, Laws, and Regulations on Medical Device Development

Japanese regulatory law concerning medical devices is mainly covered by the Pharmaceutical Affair Law and administered by the Ministry for Health, Labor, and Welfare (MHLW). The law has undergone a significant change from 1997 since the reorganization of the Drug and Medical Device Examination Center in the MHLW to bring the systems into line with those of the United States and Europe. Detailed discussion of this change, along with pre-market approval, quality system requirements, and postmarket surveillance, can be found in Ohashi [2].

The approval of medical devices has to go through various institutions. The final approval process is carried out the Drug and Medical Device Examination Center (DMDEC) in the MHLW) and the Japan Association for Advancement of Medical Equipment (JAAME).

The DMDEC was founded in July 1997 as a front end in the medical evaluation process. Currently, effort is being made to shorten the approval process to 3 years. This effort includes doubling the number of examiners and officials in the center. In addition, efforts to secure international harmonization among regulations on pharmaceuticals are being promoted, aiming to provide excellent drugs promptly to nationals, through, for example, the International Conference on Harmonization (ICH) of Technical Requirements for the Registration of Pharmaceuticals for Human Use among Japan, the US and the EU. See Fujiwara [3] for physicians' perspectives on the newly established DMDEC.

Appointed by the Minister for Health, Labor, and Welfare as the designated agency under Paragraph 3, Article 14, of the Pharmaceutical Affairs Law, the main role of the JAAME in the regulatory process is to examine the structures and performance of the medical devices submitted for approval, based on the Pharmaceutical Affairs Law, and to assess their equivalence to medical devices previously approved.

In the evaluation process, the JAAME checks the structure, intended use, efficacy, effectiveness, performance, and other factors of medical devices for which an application for approval of manufacturing or import has been submitted in order to determine its equivalency to products that have already obtained manufacturing or import approval as medical devices.

The JAAME is also engaged in promotion of the development of the medical-device industry and strengthening the health of the people and the progress of medical studies.

Standards for the Implementation of Clinical Trials of Drugs

An initiative taken by the MHLW to promote safe, lawful, and ethical clinical trials is the Standards on the Implementation of Clinical Trials on Drugs, or New GCO, enacted in April 1998. Efforts for the smooth implementation of clinical examinations are also being promoted, including the establishment of a system to invite positive participation of subjects in clinical examinations and improvement of a system of medical institutions conducting clinical examinations. This is done to activate clinical examinations in Japan, which have reportedly become stagnant. Based on the new GCO, medical institutions and their internal review boards conducting clinical trials oversee the trials.

Translational Research Center

An initiative taken by the Ministry of Education, Culture, Sports, Science, and Technology (MEXT) is the Translational Research Center, which mainly funds national universities to support scientific and clinical developments in medicine. The goal of the program is to establish a smooth transition of research and development from the laboratory stage through preclinical trials, regulatory approval, and eventually to clinical trials.

Multidisciplinary Collaborative Research Initiative

Industry, clinical institutions, and scientists have important roles in the development of medical devices. Recognizing this importance, the Ministry of Economy, Trade, and Industry (METI) has initiated an effort to promote medical device development involving multidisciplinary sectors. The steering government agency administrating the projects is the New Energy and Industrial Technology Development Organization (NEDO). The first project described below is the National Research and Development Program for Medical and Welfare Apparatus, mainly supporting the medical-device industry. The second project is the Fundamental Research Program for Advanced Medical Apparatus Undertaken in Cooperation with Medical and Engineering Researchers, or the Medical and Engineering Collaborative Research Program.

TABLE 1. Projects in the National Research and Development Program for Medical and Welfare Apparatus by NEDO and METI (as of 2001)

Medical devices
  Microanalysis system of cell information
  Graphical analyzer for human chromosomes using a confocal laser scanning microscope
  Intravascular 3D ultrasound imaging system for supporting less invasive diagnosis
  Ultrasonic treatment system
  High-speed and three-dimensional CT using a cone beam x-ray
  Unified support system for diagnosis and treatment of heart disease
  Computer-assisted analysis system for medicinal compound screening
  Acoustical dynamic 3D imaging system for medical diagnosis
  Ultrasonic-based tissue characterization system for arterial wall treatment
  Microangiographic system using quasi-monochromatic x-ray radiation
  Advanced support system for endoscopic and other minimally invasive surgery
  Totally implantable artificial heart for clinical use
  Implantable insulin infusion system utilizing optical blood glucose monitor welfare field
Welfare devices
  Home rehabilitation support system for aphasia
  Rehabilitation system upper and lower limbs
  Intelligent-assist function
  Real time sensing system
  Support system for seniors
  Daily life support system for elderly

National Research and Development Program for Medical and Welfare Apparatus

The National Research and Development Program for Medical and Welfare Apparatus targets the development of high-performance, low-cost medical and welfare equipment. Research projects are mainly conducted by the private sector applying new industrial technologies. As of 2001, 46 projects have been completed and 17 projects are active. Numerous products have been commercialized from the program. As of fiscal year 1999, 51 projects had been completed (Table 1).

Fundamental Research Program for Advanced Medical Apparatus Undertaken in Cooperation with Medical and Engineering Researchers

The second project, the Fundamental Research Program for Advanced Medical Apparatus Undertaken in Cooperation with Medical and Engineering Researchers, or the Medical and Engineering Collaborative Research Program, is intended to support medical device development and research by funding medical and engineering schools. The supporting agency, NEDO, believes that breaking the conceptual, or sometimes the language, barrier between medical and

TABLE 2. Projects in Fundamental Research Program for Advanced Medical Apparatus Undertaken in Cooperation with Medical and Engineering Researchers, by NEDO and METI (as of 2001)

Project	Period	Institution
New diagnostic and treatment system for cardiovascular disease	10–14	Tokyo University
Sensitive molecular diagnosis system for early detection of potential cancer patients using plasma DNA analysis	10–13	Okayama University
Fundamental research for minimally invasive/ super selective local diagnosis and treatment	10–15	Keio University
Fundamental research for an MRI diagnosis and treatment system	11–15	Institute of Biomedical Research and Innovation
Fundamental research for a highly effective sectional imaging system using optical interference	12–15	Yamagata University
Fundamental research for a DNA sensory system using a modified DNA electrode array	12–14	Tsukuba University

engineering researchers is critical for the efficient development of medical devices. Therefore, the main objective of the program is to bring multidisciplinary researchers and clinicians to the program to facilitate communication and collaborative work. As of 2001, six universities have been funded to conduct mainly medical device development. (Table 2)

References

1. Rogers A (1997) European drug industry concerned over proposed clinical-trial legislation. Lancet North Am Ed 350(9091):1609
2. Ohashi J (1998) Marketing medical devices in Japan. Med Device Technol 9(1):32–33, 36–37
3. Fujiwara Y (1998) MD reviewers' role in the new anticancer drug approval process in the newly established Japanese regulatory agency, PMDEC (Pharmaceuticals and Medical Devices Evaluation Center). Jpn J Clin Oncol 28(11): 653–656

Clinical Practice Guideline for Benign Prostate Hyperplasia in Japan

Yoshihiko Hirao[1], Yoshinari Ono[2], and Momokazu Gotoh[2]

Summary. The Japanese Clinical Practice Guideline for Benign prostate Hyperplasia was established in March 1999. The 1999 Guideline was developed according to the methodology of evidence-based medicine by a panel consisting of 10 academic and 10 practicing urologists and 2 epidemiologists, in cooperation with the Japanese Urological Association. The 1999 Guideline consisted of diagnostic and treatment sections. Diagnosis is made according to the International Prostate Symptom Score (I-PSS), the quality-of-life (QOL) score, the maximal flow rate on uroflowmetry, the volume of residual urine, and the estimated prostate volume by ultrasonography. According to the severity of disease, patients are classified into three categories: mild, moderate, and severe. The treatment modalities are watchful waiting, medication, minimal invasive therapy, and surgery. "Mild" patients are recommended to select either watchful waiting or medication; "moderate" patients choose medication, minimal invasive therapy, or surgery; and "severe" patients are recommended to undergo minimal invasive therapy on surgery. The background for the development of the 1999 Guideline is also described.

Key Words. Benign prostate hyperplasia, Clinical practice guideline, Evidence-based medicine

Introduction

The purpose of a clinical practice guideline is to define the most effective methods for diagnosing diseases and to identify and describe their most appropriate treatment modalities based on patient preference and clinical need. Clinical practice guidelines should provide the best diagnostic procedure and treatment modality for each patient in such aspects as medicine, cost, and quality of life. Clinical practice guidelines were first established by authority, but they

[1] Department of Urology, Nara Prefectural Medical University, 840 Shijo-cho, Kashihara, Nara 634-0813, Japan
[2] Department of Urology, Nagoya University Graduate School of Medicine, 65 Tsurumai-cho, Showa-ku, Nagoya 466-8550, Japan

were not widely used in clinical practice. They were then established by a panel of authorities, but clinical practice was still not standardized. In Japan, after a series of false starts to standardize practice, clinical guidelines have now been successfully established from evidence-based medicine by panels consisting of physicians, surgeons, nurses, other health-care professionals, and patients. These guidelines are well known to standardize clinical practice and reduce medical costs. They also help clinicians in decision making, since the increasing volume of health-care information has become too great for evaluation and use in clinical practice.

Benign prostate hyperplasia (BPH) is one of the most common urological diseases in Japan. Six hundred thousand men were diagnosed with BPH in 1998; the cost in 1997 was 148 billion yen, nearly 5% of the total expenditure for health care. Moreover, medical costs are expected to increase explosively in the next decade as the aging male population increases.

The first reason for establishing clinical practice guidelines for this condition is the variability of patient preferences for treatment. For example, significant variations exist in the individual patient's perceptions of the difficulties and risks of treatment for BPH, which is primarily a quality-of-life disease with a low mortality rate. Since the patient should play a significant role in determining his treatment, the diagnostic procedures, the treatment modalities, and the decision-making process should be clearly described and easily understood by physicians, surgeons, and nurses so that a caring health-care professional can work together with the patient to decide on optimal treatment. The second reason for the establishment of clinical practice guidelines is that a variety of diagnostic procedures and treatment modalities are employed in clinical practice for patients with BPH, with each urologist using his or her own preferred methods. In other words, diagnostic procedures and treatment modalities are different for every urologist. Such discrepancies are even wider among non-urologists. Cost is the third reason why clinical practice guidelines for BPH should be established.

Clinical Practice Guidelines for BPH Established in 1999

The Japanese Ministry of Health and Welfare planned to develop clinical practice guidelines for some common diseases in the late 1990s. The authors received a grant from the ministry in 1999 and organized a committee to develop clinical practice guidelines for urological diseases. The committee, consisting of three academic urologists, two practicing urologists, and two epidemiologists, selected BPH and female incontinence for the development of the guidelines, because both diseases are benign and significantly influence quality of life; patients are treated with various modalities ranging from medication to surgery; patients are treated by urologists and non-urologists, such as gynecologists and family practitioners; and the outcome of clinical practice guidelines can be easily evaluated.

Grand Design

Clinical practice guidelines are developed according to methods provided by evidence-based medicine. The panel members appointed by the committee included ten academic urologists, ten practicing urologists, two epidemiologists, the chairman of the executive committee of the Japanese Society of Urology, and officers of the Ministry of Health and Welfare. The grand design included establishment of structure and definition of research subjects, critical appraisal of the literature, economic assessment, development of clinical practice guidelines, and assessment of clinical guidelines and their renewal.

Establishment of Structure and Definition of Research Subjects

In developing clinical practice guidelines, a standard patient with the target disease is postulated. In the guideline for patients with BPH, the standard patient was defined as a man at least 50 years old complaining of difficulty in urinating and being treated with modalities as described in the clinical practice guideline. According to the severity of disease, patients were divided into three subgroups: mild, moderate, and severe. The conventional treatment modalities for each subgroup were listed. Treatment modalities not covered by insurance were omitted from the list for practical use.

The research subjects were chosen to evaluate the efficacy of each listed treatment modality and to compare the results in each subgroup. The most appropriate modality was then determined for each subgroup.

Critical Appraisal of the Literature

Clinical practice guidelines for BPH have been published previously by the American Urological Association [1] and the World Health Organization and Agency for Health Research and Quality [2], among others, and, along with the National Guideline Clearinghouse, have a database of manuscripts. However, 411 manuscripts indicated by both "treatment" and "benign prostate hyperplasia" were independently found in the Cochran Library and Medline between 1989 and 1999. All 411 manuscripts underwent critical appraisal by all members, and evaluations of 390 manuscripts were done. The impact of each manuscript on the clinical practice guideline was defined according to the criteria shown in Fig. 1. The recommendable grade for each manuscript was defined as shown in Table 1. Forty-five manuscripts ultimately were adopted in the clinical practice guideline [2–46].

Economic Assessment

Treatment modalities with proven efficacy should be assessed economically in developing clinical practice guidelines. However, economic assessment was not

First Author		Country		Published Year	
Journal				Vol. Page ~	
Purpose					
	☐Randomized	☐Nonrandomized		☐Intent-to-treat analysis	
Patients	Total number:	Mild · Moderate · Severe · Unknown			
Treatment modality	A:	: Number			
	B:	: Number			
	C:	: Number			
Results	A		B		C
	Baseline → Final		Baseline → Final		Baseline → Final
IPSS	→ *		→ *		→ *
QOL	→ *		→ *		→ *
Q_{max}	→ *		→ *		→ *
Residual volume	→ *		→ *		→ *
Other					
Adverse effect					
Statistics					
Observation period		Rate of dropout			
Conclusion					
Assessment	I · II · III · IV · V				

FIG. 1. Assessment list: clinical study of BPH treatment

TABLE 1. Levels of evidence for evaluation of antithrombotic agents [47]

Level I: Randomized trial with low false-positive and false-negative errors (high power)
Level II: Randomized trial with high false-positive and/or high false-negative errors (low power)
Level III: Non-randomized concurrent cohort comparisons between patients who did and did not receive both antithrombotic agents
Level IV: Non-randomized historical cohort comparisons between current patients who did receive antithrombotic agents and former patients (from the same institution or from the literature) who did not
Level V: Case series without control subjects

performed in the 1999 Guideline because there were few manuscripts indicating the cost of treatment modalities for BPH or the long-term effectiveness of treatment modalities in Japan. These data are necessary to determine the cost-effectiveness of various treatment modalities and will be available in the outcome research of the 1999 Clinical Practice Guideline.

Development of Clinical Practice Guideline

The 1999 Clinical Practice Guideline was developed mainly from the 45 manuscripts [2–46] by four panel members, and was then reviewed and corrected by all panel members. It is necessary for the 1999 Guideline to be further reviewed and corrected by physicians, surgeons, family practitioners, nurses, other health care professionals, officers, and patients.

Assessment of Clinical Guideline and Its Renewal

Assessment of the 1999 Clinical Guideline is proceeding in 2001 and 2002. It will consist of evaluation of compliance with the guideline; its availability to patients; treatment efficacy based on uroflowmetry, residual volume, International Prostate Symptom Score (I-PSS), and quality-of-life (QOL) score; and the total cost for patient care and cost-effectiveness analysis. Renewal will also be planned in 2003.

Contents of Clinical Practice Guideline for BPH

Clinical decisions concerning the diagnosis and treatment of BPH patients proceed in accordance with the algorithm for standard clinical practice (Fig. 2).

Diagnosis

Because BPH is not a life-threatening disease but rather has a significant impact on patients' QOL, the evaluation of subjective symptoms and impact on QOL

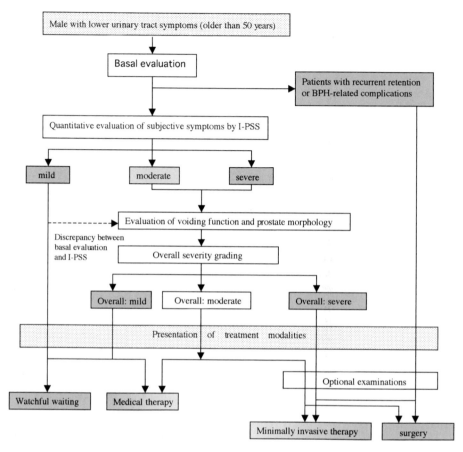

Fig. 2. Algorithm for standard diagnosis and treatment of benign prostate hyperplasia (BPH), I-PSS, International Prostate Symptom Score

based on patients' perspective is of primary importance in evaluating the severity of the disease [3].

According to this guideline, a patient complaining of lower urinary tract symptoms (LUTS) undergoes basal diagnostic evaluation. When the basal evaluation is suggestive of voiding dysfunction, an assessment of subjective symptoms by the I-PSS is performed. Moderate or severe I-PSS scores call for further evaluation of objective findings of voiding function and prostate morphology. The overall severity of the disease is graded based on the four domains of subjective symptoms, QOL, voiding function, and prostate morphology.

Basal Diagnostic Evaluation [4]

All patients complaining of LUTS undergo the following basal evaluation.

Medical History

Interview focusing on general health status, voiding status, previous surgical procedures, current medications, and other disorders possibly affecting voiding function.

Physical Examinations

Digital rectal examination and neurological examination.

Urine Examination

Urinalysis by either dipstick or microscopic examination of sediment.

Serum Creatinine

Prostate Specific Antigen (PSA) (Optional)

Although measurement of serum PSA level is optional, it is more sensitive for the detection of prostate cancer than digital rectal examination and is recommended to be included in the basal examination [5].

In the present guideline, patients with specific conditions, such as recurrent or persistent episodes of urinary retention or macrohematuria, bladder stones, or impaired renal function, are categorized as having serious BPH, independently of the algorithm. These patients need urgent and radical treatment, usually by surgery.

Quantitative Evaluation of Subjective Symptoms by I-PSS

Subjective symptoms of BPH are quantitatively assessed by using I-PSS and QOL scores (Fig. 3). The I-PSS consists of seven items, each of which is scored from 0 to 5. The total I-PSS score is calculated by adding the scores of each item, and it ranges from 0 to 35. The severity of subjective symptoms is graded from mild (0 to 7 of I-PSS) to moderate (8 to 19), to severe (20 to 35) [4,6]. The QOL score is categorized in seven grades according to patient satisfaction with voiding status, from 0 (very satisfied) to 7 (very unsatisfied) [4,6].

Patients with moderate to severe I-PSS undergo further objective evaluation of voiding function and prostate morphology.

Evaluation of Voiding Function and Prostate Morphology

Evaluation of voiding function includes uroflowmetry and measurement of residual urine volume. Prostate morphology is assessed in terms of prostate volume measured by ultrasonography. These examinations are important objective evaluations and are employed in grading the severity of BPH, deciding treatment options, and assessing treatment efficacy [4,7].

Voiding Function

Uroflowmetry provides an objective and quantitative evaluation of voiding condition in a less invasive fashion [8,11], with the maximum flow rate (Q_{max}) in

I-PSS

Questions	Not at all	Less than 1 time in 5	Less than half the time	About half the time	More than half the time	Almost always
1. Over the past month, how often have you had a sensation of not emptying your bladder completely after you finished urinating	0	1	2	3	4	5
2. Over the past month, how often have you had to urinate again less than 2 hours after you finished urinating?	0	1	2	3	4	5
3. Over the past month, how often have you found you stopped and started again several times when you urinated?	0	1	2	3	4	5
4. Over the past month, how often have you found it difficult to postpone urination?	0	1	2	3	4	5
5. Over the past month, how often have you had a weak urinary stream?	0	1	2	3	4	5
6. Over the past month, how often have you had to push or strain to begin urination?	0	1	2	3	4	5
7. Over the past month, how many times did you most typically get up to urinate from the time you went to bed at night until the time you got up in the morning?	0 (None)	1 (1 time)	2 (2 times)	3 (3 times)	4 (4 times)	5 (5 times or more)

Sum of 7 circled numbers (I-PSS)

Quality of life score

	Delighted	Pleased	Mostly satisfied	Mixed about equally satisfied and dissatisfied	Mostly dissatisfied	Unhappy	Terrible
1. If you were to spend the rest of your life with your urinary condition just the way it is now, how would you feel about that?							

FIG. 3. International Prostate Symptom Score (I-PSS)

milliliters per second being a parameter of primary importance. Uroflowmetry, however, is of little use in distinguishing between bladder outlet obstruction and impaired detrusor contraction. A pressure-flow study is a more appropriate examination for that purpose.

Measurement of residual urine is performed by transurethral catheterization or, preferably, by less invasive transabdominal ultrasonography [12]. Because the reproducibility of residual urine measurement is low, repeated measurements should be taken [13]. It is to be elucidated whether residual urine volume can predict treatment efficacy.

Voiding dysfunction is graded from mild (Q_{max} ≥15 ml/s and residue <50 ml), to moderate (Q_{max} ≥5 ml/s and residue <100 ml), to severe (Q_{max} <5 ml/s or residue ≥100 ml) [4,6].

Prostate Morphology

Prostate morphology is evaluated as prostate volume (milliliters) by either transrectal or transabdominal ultrasonography. Although transrectal ultrasonography needs specific equipment, it provides clearer visualization of prostate structures and more detailed observation of prostate morphology. Prostate volume can also be measured by the presence of urine inside the bladder on transabdominal ultrasonography [14–17].

Ultrasonography visualizes the prostate in two dimensions, usually by cross and longitudinal sections. Prostate volume can be calculated by multiplying the three dimensions of the visualized prostate and dividing by 2 (volume = length × height × width/2 ml).

Enlargement of prostate volume is graded from mild (<20 ml) to moderate (<50 ml) to severe (≥50 ml).

Overall Severity Grading

The overall severity is graded from mild to moderate to severe based on the severity of each domain: I-PSS, QOL, voiding function, and prostate morphology. The severity grading of each domain is summarized in Table 2. The overall severity is determined by the numbers of severity grades of each domain (Table 3). This grading system is according to the guideline included in the Clinical Trial Guideline for Voiding Dysfunction edited by the Japanese Urological Association [6].

TABLE 2. Severity grading criteria for each domain

Severity	Symptoms I-PSS	QOL score	Voiding function Q_{max} and residue	Prostate volume (ml)
Mild	0–7	0, 1	≧15 ml/s and <50 ml	<20
Moderate	8–19	2, 3, 4	≧5 ml/s and <100 ml	<50
Severe	20–35	5, 6	<5 ml/s or ≧100 ml	≧50

I-PSS, International Prostate Symptom Score; QOL, quality of life.

TABLE 3. Criteria for overall severity grading

Overall severity	Numbers of each severity grade in 4 domains		
	Mild	Moderate	Severe
Mild	4	0	0
	3	1	0
Moderate	Any	$\geqq 2$	0
	Any	Any	1
Severe	Any	Any	$\geqq 2$

Optional Examinations to Decide the Indication of Surgery

Pressure-Flow Study

A pressure-flow study distinguishes between bladder outlet obstruction and impaired detrusor contraction, although the procedure is somewhat invasive. A pressure-flow study provides a quantitative evaluation of the grade of obstruction and detrusor function and useful information to predict treatment efficacy. When causes of voiding dysfunction other than bladder outlet obstruction are suspected, such as in patients with diabetic peripheral neuropathy or small prostates, it is advisable to perform a pressure-flow study to decide treatment options [18,19].

Urethrocystoscopy

Urethrocystoscopy provides detailed observation of the inside of the bladder and the prostatic urethra. Although it is an invasive examination, it may be useful to determine surgical treatment [20].

Examinations Unnecessary for Diagnosis of BPH

Morphological Evaluation of the Upper Urinary Tract

For patients with mild to moderate BPH, imaging of the upper urinary tract by either excretory urography or ultrasonography is unnecessary. These examinations are indicated for patients with complicated urinary tract disorders or episodes of macrohematuria, persistent urinary tract infection, renal failure, recurrent urinary retention, or urinary tract stones [21,22].

Retrograde Urethrocystography

Retrograde urethrocystography is invasive and of little diagnostic value, but it may play some role in the diagnosis of urethral stenosis when it is suspected [23,24].

Filling Cystometry

Cystometry provides information only on the storage function of the bladder. The diagnostic value in BPH is lower than that of a pressure-flow study [25]. Filling cystometry is not recommended for routine use.

Treatment

BPH patients with minimal subjective symptoms rarely need treatment, whereas surgical treatment is an appropriate choice for those with BPH-related complications. Otherwise, because BPH is a QOL disease, the physician should decide a treatment option based on informed consent, discussing with the patient the purpose of the treatment, its efficacy, possible complications of each treatment modality, and any other problems.

At present, the treatment modality for BPH is divided into five categories: watchful waiting, medical therapy, minimally invasive therapy, surgery, and indwelling catheter.

Watchful Waiting

It has been demonstrated that one quarter of patients with mild to moderate BPH will have a spontaneous improvement in voiding dysfunction [26]. Watchful waiting should be a standard option of management for patients with mild BPH.

Medical Therapy

Medical therapy is indicated for patients with mild to moderate BPH.

Alpha-Adrenoceptor Blocking Agents

Alpha-blockers decrease urethral resistance and improve voiding dysfunction by relaxing the smooth muscle of the prostate and bladder neck. A variety of alpha-blockers selective to alpha 1-receptor subtypes have been developed to improve drug efficacy and decrease adverse effects, such as orthotopic hypotension and dizziness [27–30]. The appearance of the drug effect is rather prompt after administration, and its efficacy lasts for a long period. Alpha-blockers are standard therapy among medical treatments for BPH patients.

Antiandrogen Drugs

Hormonal therapy with antiandrogen drugs improves prostatic obstruction by reducing the size of the prostate [31–33]. The appearance of clinical efficacy is slow, and discontinuation of administration causes regrowth of the prostate. The adverse effects of the antiandrogen therapy are those associated with sexual function, such as decreased sexual desire and erectile dysfunction.

Because antiandrogen administration decreases the serum PSA level, it should be kept in mind that long-term hormonal treatment may interfere with the detection of complicated prostate cancer [34]. The efficacy of combined use of alpha-blockers and antiandrogen has yet to be elucidated because of a lack of clinical trials [35].

Other Drugs

Plant extracts, amino acid complexes, and herbal medicines have been used for treatment of BPH. However, the mechanisms of action and the efficacy of these drugs are still to be elucidated [36].

Minimally Invasive Therapies

This category of modern treatments includes laser, stent, and thermal therapies. Although a number of papers have reported the lack of invasiveness and the safety of these treatments, there is still a lack of studies confirming their long-term efficacy as compared with conventional therapies [37–43]. Further clinical trials are necessary for these treatment modalities to be recognized as standard. Because these treatment modalities are expected to play a more important role in the management of BPH in the future, further randomized clinical trials are needed.

Surgery

Surgical treatment is indicated for patients with moderate to severe overall severity or with BPH-related complications. Among a variety of treatment modalities for BPH, surgery is the most invasive but also the most effective for improvement of bladder outlet obstruction. Although open prostatectomy may be performed in patients with an excessively large prostate, it is more invasive and has a higher risk of operative complications than TURP (transurethral resection of prostate). TURP is a well-established procedure that is the gold standard for the surgical treatment of BPH [45,46].

Indwelling Urethral Catheter

Transurethral placement of a Foley catheter may be useful for temporary management of urinary retention. However, because long-term placement of an indwelling catheter is associated with urinary tract complications and impairs the patient's QOL, definitive treatment, such as surgery, should be considered in patients with chronic urinary retention. Clean intermittent catheterization performed by caregivers or patients is a well-established and safe procedure.

Acknowledgement. The 1999 Japanese Clinical Practice Guideline for benign prostate hyperplasia was developed by the grant from The Japanese Ministry of Health and Labor.

References

1. U.S. Department of Health and Human Services, Agency for Health Care Policy and Research (1994) Clinical Practice Guideline; Benign Prostatic Hyperplasia; Diagnosis
2. Cockett ATK, Khoury S, Aso Y, Chatelain C, Denis L, Griffiths K, Murphy (eds) (1995) Proceedings of the 3rd International Consultation on Benign Prostatic Hyperplasia (BPH) (level V)
3. Berry SJ, Coffey DS, Walsh PC, Ewing LL (1984) The development of human benign prostatic hyperplasia with age. J Urol 132:474–479 (level V)
4. Koyanagi T, Artibani W, Correa R, Desgranchamps F, DeReijke TM, Govier F, Hanash K, Hirano Y, Hoisaeter PA, Kobayashi S, Kurth KH, Marshall VR, Palmtag H, Wasserman N, Zerbib M (1999) Initial diagnostic evaluation of men with lower urinary tract symptoms. In: Proceedings of the 4th International Consultation on Benign Prostatic hyperplasia (BPH) (level V)
5. Oesterling JE, Jacobson SJ, Cooner WH (1995) The use of age-specific reference ranges for serum prostatic antigen in men 60 years old or older. J Urol 153:1160–1163 (level V)
6. Panel for Clinical Trial Guideline on Voiding Dysfunction (1997) Clinical trial guideline on voiding dysfunction. Igaku Tosho Shuppan Tokyo (level V)
7. Kaplan SA, Olsson CA, Te AE (1996) The American Urological Association symptom score in the evaluation of men with lower urinary tract symptoms; at 2 years of followup. Does it work? J Urol 144:1974–1974 (level III)
8. Halt T (1989) Urodynamics in benign prostatic hyperplasia; a survey. Prostate (suppl) 2:69–77 (level IV)
9. Poulson A, Schou J, Puggaard L, Torp-Pedersen S, Nordling J (1994) Prostatic enlargement, symptomatology and pressure/flow evaluation; interrelation in patients with symptomatic BPH. Scand J Urol Nephrol Suppl 157:67–73 (level V)
10. Mah P, Lim C, Abrams Z, Abrams P (1995) Are urine flow studies adequate for the investigation of older men with lower urinary tract symptoms? Proceedings of the 25th Annual ICS Meeting, Sydney (level V)
11. De la Rosette JJMCM, Witjes WPJ, Debruyne FMY, Kersten PL, Wijkstre H (1996) Improved reliability of uroflowmetry investigation; results of a portable home-based uroflowmetry study. Br J Urol 78:385–390 (level IV)
12. Roehborn CG, Chinn HK, Fulgham PF, Simpkins KL, Peters PC (1986) The role of transabdominal ultrasound in the preoperative evaluation of patients with benign prostatic hypertrophy. J Urol 135:1190–1193 (level V)
13. Barry MJ, Cockett AT, Holtgrewe HL, Mcxconnell JD, Sihelnik SA, Winfield HN (1993) Relationship of symptoms of prostatism to commonly used physiological and anatomical measures of the severity of benign prostatic hyperplasia. J Urol 150:351–358 (level IV)
14. Bosch JLHR, Kranse R, van Mastrungt R, Schroder FH (1995) Reasons for the weak correlation between prostate volume and urethral resistance parameters in patients with prostatism. J Urol 153:689–693 (level III)
15. Kaplan SA, Te AE, Pressler LB, Olsson CA (1993) Transition zone index (TZI) as a method of assessing benign prostatic hyperplasia; correlation with symptoms, uroflow and detrusor pressure. J Urol 154:1764–1769 (level V)
16. Hough DM, List A (1991) Reliability of transabdominal ultrasound in the measurement of prostate size. Aust Radiol 35:358–360 (level V)

17. Bangma CH, Niemer AQHJ, Grobbee DE, Schroder FH (1996) Transrectal ultrasonic volumetry of the prostate; in vivo comparison of different methods. Prostate 28: 107–110 (level V)
18. Gerber CS (1996) The role of urodynamic study in the evaluation and management of men with lower urinary tract symptoms secondary to benign prostatic hyperplasia. Urology 48:668–675 (level V)
19. McConnel JD (1994) Why pressure-flow studies should be optional and not mandatory studies for evaluating men with benign prostatic hyperplasia. Urology 44:156–158 (level V)
20. El Din KE, De Wildt MJAM, Rosier PFWM, Debruyne FMJ, De la Rosette JJMCH (1996) The correlation between urodynamics and cystoscopic findings in elderly men with voiding complaints. J Urol 155:1018–1022 (level V)
21. Kock WFRM, El Din KE, De Wildt MJAM, Debruyne FMJ, De La Rosette JJMCH (1996) The outcome of renal ultrasound in the assessment of 556 consecutive patients with benign prostatic hyperplasia. J Urol 155:186–189 (level V)
22. Wasserman NF, Lapointe S, Eckmann DR, Rosel PR (1987) Assessment of prostatism; role of intravenous urography. Radiology 165:831–835 (level V)
23. Aguirre CR, Tallada MB, Mayayo TD, Perales LC, Romero JM (1980) Comparative evaluation of prostate size by transabdominal echography, urethral profile and radiology. J Urol (Paris) 86(9):675–679 (level III)
24. Koyanagi T (1974) Diagnostic value of voiding cystourethrography. Jpn J Urol 65: 29–43 (level V)
25. Ameda K, Koyanagi T, Nantani M, Taniguchi K, Matsuno T (1994) The relevance of preoperative cystometrography in patients with benign prostatic hyperplasia; correlating the findings with clinical features and outcome after prostatectomy. J Urol 152:443–447 (level V)
26. Wasson JH, Reda DJ, Bruskewitz RC, Elinson J, Keller AM, Henderson WG (1995) A comparison of transurethral surgery with watchful waiting for moderate symptoms of benign prostatic hyperplasia. The Veterans Affairs Cooperative Study Group on Transurethral Resection of the Prostate. N Engl J Med 332:75–79 (level I)
27. Buzelin JM, Roth S, Geffriaud-Ricouard C, Delauche-Cavallier MC, and the ALGEBI Study Group (1996) Efficacy and safety of sustained-release alfuzosin 5 mg in patients with benign prostatic hyperplasia. Urology 47:335–342 (level I)
28. Roehborn CG, Oesterling JE, Auerbach S, Kaplan SA, Lloyd LK, Milam DR, et al. for the HYCAT Investigator Group (1996) The Hytrin Community Assessment Trial Study; one-year study of terazosin versus placebo in the treatment of men with symptomatic benign prostatic hyperplasia. Urology 47:139–168 (level I)
29. Roherborn CG, Siegel RL (1996) Safety and efficacy of doxazosin in benign prostatic hyperplasia; a pooled analysis of three double-blind, placebo-controlled studies. Urology 48:406–415 (level I)
30. Chapple CR, Wyndaele JJ, Nordling J, Boeminghaus F, Ypma AFGVM, Abrams P (1996) Tamsulosin, the first prostate-selective alpha 1A-adrenoceptor antagonist; a meta-analysis of two randomized, placebo-controlled, multicentre studies in patients with benign prostatic obstruction (symptomatic BPH). Eur Urol 29:155–167 (level I)
31. En LM, Tveter KJ (1993) A prospective, placebo-controlled study of luteinizing hormone-releasing hormone agonist leuprolide as treatment for patients with benign prostatic hyperplasia. J Urol 150:359–364 (level I)
32. Shida K (1986) Clinical effects of allylestrenol on benign prostatic hypertrophy by double-blind method. Acta Urol Jpn 32:625–648 (level I)

33. Stoner E, the Finasteride Study Group (1994) Three-year safety and efficacy data on the use of finasteride in the treatment of benign prostatic hyperplasia. Urology 43: 284–294 (level I)

34. Stoner E, the Finasteride Study Group (1994) Clinical experience of the detection of prostate cancer in patients with benign prostatic hyperplasia treated with finasteride. J Urol 151:1296–1300 (level I)

35. Lepor H, Williford WO, Barry MJ, Brawer MK, Dixon CM, Gormley G, Haakenson C, Machi M, Narayan P, Padley RJ, for the Veterans Affairs Cooperative Studies Benign Prostatic Hyperplasia Study Group (1996) The efficacy of terazosin, finasteride, or both in benign prostatic hyperplasia. N Engl J Med 335:533–539 (level I)

36. Dreikorn K, Borkowski A, Braeckman J, Denis L, Ferrari P, Gerber G, Levin R, Lowe F, Perrin P, Senge T (1997) Other medical therapies. In: Proceedings of the 4th International Consultation on Benign Prostatic Hyperplasia, pp 663–659 (level V)

37. Cowles RS III, Kabalin JN, Childs S, Lepor H, Dixon C, Stein BS, Zabbo A (1995) A prospective randomized comparison of transurethral resection to visual laser ablation of the prostate for the treatment of benign prostatic hyperplasia. Urology 46:155 (level II)

38. Whilfield HN (1996) A randomized prospective multicenter study evaluating the efficacy of interstitial laser coagulation. J Urol 155:318A (level II)

39. Muschter R (1996) Interstitial laser therapy. Curr Opinion Urol 6:33–38 (level III)

40. Chapple CR, Rosario DJ, Wasserfaallen M, Woo HH, Nordling J, MiLroy EJG (1995) A randomized study of the Urolume stent vs prostatic surgery. J Urol 153 (suppl): 436A (level II)

41. Dahlstrand C, Walden M, Geirsson G, Pettersson S (1993) Transurethral microwave thermotherapy versus transurethral resection for symptomatic benign prostatic obstruction; a prospective randomized study with a 2-year follow-up. Br J Urol 76:614 (level II)

42. De la Rosette J, Tubaro A, Trucehi A, Carter SSTC, Hofner K (1995) Changes in pressure flow parameters in patients treated by transurethral microwave thermotherapy using Prostasoft 2.0. J Urol 154:1382 (level I)

43. Oesterling JE, Arbor A, Muta MI, Roehrborn CG, Perez-Marrero R, Bruskewitz R, Madison WI, Naslund MJ, Shumaker BP, Perinchary N (1997) A single blind, prospective randomized clinical trial comparing transurethral needle ablation (TUNA) to transurethral resection of the prostate (TURP) for the treatment of benign prostatic hyperplasia (BPH). J Urol 157:A1282 (level II)

44. Nakamura K (1996) Treatment of BPH (benign prostatic hypertrophy); high intensity focused ultrasound (HIFU). Curr Ther 14(11): 1–6 (level IV)

45. Holtgrewe HL, Mebust WK, Dowd JB, Cockett ATK, Peters PC, Proctor C (1989) Transurethral prostatectomy; practice aspects of the dominant operation in American urology. J Urol 141:248–253 (level V)

46. Rechmann M, Knes JA, Neisey D, Madsen PO, Bruskewitz RC (1995) Transurethral resection versus incision of the prostate; a randomized, prospective study. Urology 145:768–775 (level II)

47. Cook DJ, et al. (1992) Rules of evidence and clinical recommendations on the use of antithrombotic agents. Chest 102:3050–3056

Standard Treatment Modality for Ureteral Calculi

MATTHEW T. GETTMAN and CLAUS G. ROEHRBORN

Summary. Technological advances have significantly impacted the treatment of ureteral calculi. A variety of minimally invasive alternatives are available to treat ureteral calculi. Despite the development of practice guidelines, considerable controversy surrounds the optimal choice of treatment for ureteral calculi.

Key Words. Ureteroscopy, Shock-wave lithotripsy, Surgical treatment, ureteral calculus, Percutaneous nephrostolithotomy, Laparoscopy

Introduction

Technological advances and physician innovation have improved the treatment of ureteral calculi. Shock-wave lithotripsy (SWL) and ureteroscopy (URS) are the most common first-line treatments for ureteral calculi. Percutaneous nephrostolithotomy (PCNL) is occasionally recommended, primarily for treatment of proximal ureteral stones. Open and laparoscopic ureterolithotomy are exceedingly rare as first-line treatments. Despite favorable outcomes with a variety of minimally invasive modalities, optimal treatment remains controversial in certain instances [1].

The majority of patients with symptoms of renal colic will spontaneously pass their ureteral stones. The likelihood of spontaneous passage is influenced by stone size and location. In their series of 520 patients, Ueno and associates evaluated the frequency of spontaneous stone passage and found an overall rate of 55%. They noted that for stones measuring <4 mm, 4–6 mm, and >6 mm in diameter, spontaneous stone passage was observed in 80%, 59%, and 21% of cases, respectively [2]. In a meta-analysis of 327 articles, Segura and colleagues found the likelihood of spontaneous passage to be 29%–98% (95% CI) for stones <5 mm above the iliac vessels (proximal calculi) and 71%–98% (95% CI) for

Department of Urology, University of Texas Southwestern Medical Center, 5323 Harry Hines Blvd. J8.130, Dallas, TX 75390-9110, USA stones below the iliac vessels (distal calculi). Passage of stones between 5 and 10 mm occurred in 10%–53% of cases for proximal calculi and 25%–53% of cases for distal calculi [1].

If conservative management is unsuccessful or contraindicated, definitive treatment must be undertaken. As treatment of stones has become easier to perform and less invasive for the patient, enthusiasm for a conservative approach has dwindled. Nonetheless, conservative management remains a viable option for appropriate stones and patients.

Management of Proximal Ureteral Stones

Shock-Wave Lithotripsy

Proximal ureteral calculi are often ideally suited for SWL treatment. Although early studies recommended displacement of the stone into the renal pelvis or bypassing the stone with a ureteral stent [3–5], prospective, randomized trials have demonstrated comparable success rates for in situ versus push-back and bypass SWL [6–8]. Danuser and colleagues prospectively randomized 110 patients to in situ or push-back SWL, using a Dornier HM3, and found equivalent stone-free rates (96% in situ; 94% push-back) [7]. Albala and associates noted similar results in another prospective randomized trial comparing treatment with and without a ureteral stent using a Dornier HM3 or Siemens Lithostar [8]. Stone-free rates of 67% and 80% were obtained with the Dornier HM3 with and without stent bypass, respectively, and similar rates of 89% and 74% were noted with the Lithostar. Patients treated with a stent had significantly more voiding symptoms and a longer convalescence than those not receiving a stent [8].

Other series have noted stone-free rates of 73%–96% and retreatment rates of 0%–27% with the Dornier HM3 (Table 1) [7,9,10]. For treatment with second- and third-generation lithotripters, recent reports have noted stone-free rates of 59%–96% and retreatment rates of 11%–44% for proximal ureteral calculi (Table 1) [11–19]. In recent reports, a ureteral catheter was used for 21% of patients treated with a second- or third-generation lithotripter [11–14,18] and 46% of patients treated with the Dornier HM3. Complications such as hematoma, sepsis, ileus, and ureteral injury are exceedingly rare [11,14,17,19].

Ureteroscopy

Technological advances, such as downsizing of the flexible ureteroscopes and development of holmium:yttrium-aluminum-garnet (Ho:YAG) laser lithotripsy, have greatly improved the efficiency of upper-tract stone treatment [20–30]. Improvements in balloon dilators, access sheaths, guidewires, and retrieval devices have further increased the efficiency of URS. Tawfiek and Bagley used a 7.5 F flexible ureteroscope and intracorporeal lithotripsy to successfully clear 28

TABLE 1. Results of shock wave lithotripsy (SWL) for proximal ureteral calculi using Dornier HM3 or higher-generation lithotripters

Author	Year	Lithotripter	Patients	Stone-free rate	ReTx	Aux proc.	Ureteral catheter	LOS (days)	Complications
Tiselius[a] [9]	1991	Dornier HM3	88	94% (83/88)	27% (24/88)	–	100%	–	–
Cass[a] [10]	1992	Dornier HM3	386	77% (211/273)	5% (19/386)	8% (21/273)	100% (273/273)	–	–
Cass[b] [10]	1992	Dornier HM3	478	73% (243/333)	4% (18/478)	2% (5/333)	0%	–	–
Danuser[c] [7]	1993	Dornier HM3	46	96% (44/46)	2% (1/46)	–	0%	–	–
Danuser[b] [7]	1993	Dornier HM3	48	94% (45/48)	0% (0/48)	–	0%	–	–
Subtotal	–	Dornier HM3	1046	79% (626/788)	–	–	46% (361/788)	–	–
Voce [11]	1993	MPL9000	247	96% (236/247)	20% (50/247)	5% (11/247)	9% (21/247)	–	0% (0/247)
Chang [12]	1993	Lithostar	26	77% (20/26)	33% (8/26)	8% (2/26)	0% (0/26)	–	–
Chang [12]	1993	Lithostar	27	59% (16/27)	29% (7/27)	22% (6/27)	100% (27/27)	–	–
Chang [12]	1993	Lithostar	24	63% (15/24)	44% (10/24)	21% (5/24)	100% (24/24)	–	–
Ilker [13]	1994	MFL5000	85	84% (71/85)	–	–	0% (0/84)	–	–
Frabboni [14]	1994	MPL9000	247	96% (236/247)	20% (50/247)	5% (11/247)	9% (21/247)	–	0% (0/247)
Mobley [15]	1994	Lithostar	8477	85% (4853/5719)	11%	5%	24% (1373/5719)	–	–
Grasso [16]	1995	Lithostar	27	59% (16/27)	11% (3/27)	37% (10/27)	0% (0/27)	–	–
Kupeli [17]	1998	Lithostar	458	61% (279/458)	–	–	0% (0/458)	–	3.9% (18/458)
Strohmaier [18]	1999	Modulith, Compact	38	76% (29/38)	–	24% (9/38)	39% (15/38)	–	–
Gnanapragasam [19]	1999	MFL5000	83	90% (84/93)	–	9% (8/93)	0% (0/93)	Outpatient	0% (0/93)
Subtotal	–	2nd and 3rd generation	9739	84% (5855/6991)	–	–	21% (1481/6991)	–	–

[a] Stent bypass.
[b] Pushback SWL.
[c] In situ SWL.
LOS, length of stay in hospital.

of 29 (97%) proximal ureteral calculi in a single treatment [21]. In a report by Elashry and colleagues, the newer 7.5F flexible ureteroscopes significantly decreased the need for dilation of the ureteral orifice, decreased postoperative analgesia requirements, and increased the likelihood of successful outpatient treatment [31].

One of the most important advances in endourology is the development of the Ho:YAG laser, which has made fragmentation of any stone, once accessed, a near certainty. Teichman and associates compared the fragmentation of artificial stones treated ex vivo with Ho:YAG, pulsed-dye, pneumatic, or electrohydraulic lithotripsy (EHL) and found that the Ho:YAG laser generated the smallest fragments, thereby increasing the likelihood of spontaneous passage. The authors speculated that smaller fragments would be more likely to pass after in vivo treatment [32]. Clinically, the stone-free ranges for Ho:YAG lithotripsy are 78%–99% [20,23–25,33]. However, good fragmentation and stone-free rates for proximal stones have also been reported using 1.9F EHL probes and pulsed-dye laser [34,35]. Benizri and coworkers reported a success rate of 94% (152 of 161 calculi) using pulsed-dye lithotripsy. Four of 154 patients had ureteral complications (abrasions or perforations) related to laser lithotripsy. Although safety has been a concern with larger EHL probes ($\leq$3F), Elashry and associates reported no intraoperative complications or ureteral mucosal damage during treatment of renal and ureteral calculi with 1.9F EHL probes. An overall stone-free rate of 92% was noted (32/35) at 3-month followup. The 1.9F EHL probes were more flexible and less expensive than Ho:YAG or pulsed-dye laser lithotripsy [34].

In series using smaller instruments and improved lithotrites since 1994, 66%–99% stone-free and 3%–28% secondary procedure rates are reported with URS (Table 2) [16,17,20–30]. The incidence and severity of URS complications have decreased over time [36]. For instance, the incidences of ureteral perforation and ureteral stricture were 2% and <1%, respectively, in four Ho:YAG lithotripsy series with abstractable data [20,21,23,25].

Percutaneous Surgery

PCNL constitutes first-line therapy for some large and/or impacted proximal ureteral calculi and serves as salvage therapy for others. Stone-free rates in the literature range from 88% to 100% [37–40]. PCNL of proximal ureteral calculi is associated with a complication rate of 11%–65% [37–40].

Laparoscopy

Gaur and colleagues achieved a 75% stone-free rate in 12 cases of laparoscopic ureterolithotomy for proximal ureteral calculi [41]. Three cases were converted to open ureterolithotomy after laparoscopy failed. Harewood and colleagues used a transperitoneal or retroperitoneal approach to successfully treat nine upper-tract stones. Of the three retroperitoneal attempts, two required conversion to a transperitoneal approach for successful treatment [42]. As in Gaur's

TABLE 2. Treatment of proximal ureteral stones with ureteroscopy

Author	Year	Patients	Size of ureteroscope	Modality of stone removal	Stone-free rate	LOS (days)	Complications	2nd procedure
Grasso [16]	1995	27	6.9F, 7.5F	Pulsed-dye, EHL	96% (26/27)	–	–	4% (1/27)
Jung [30]	1996	40	6.5F	Alexandrite laser	68% (27/40)	–	5% (1/40)	28% (11/40)
Yang [29]	1996	43	6.9F	EHL	84% (36/43)	2.5	9% (4/43)	14% (6/43)
Harmon [28]	1997	17	6F, 8.5F, 11.5F	Intact, EHL, USL, impactor	77% (13/17)	–	–	–
Yip [27]	1998	18	8.5F, 9.5F	Holmium:YAG	78% (14/18)	–	–	6% (1/18)
Park [26]	1998	12	7.9F–11.5F	Intact or lithoclast	75% (9/12)	–	–	–
Pearle [25]	1998	51	6.9–8.5F	Alexandrite laser	69% (35/51)	–	–	–
Kupeli [17]	1998	15	9.5F, 12F	EHL, USL, PL	66% (10/15)	–	40% (6/15)	–
Devarajan [24]	1998	114	7.5F	Holmium:YAG	88% (77/114)	–	–	11% (12/114)
Puppo [22]	1999	62	7F, 7.7F, 8F	EHL, PL	99% (61/62)	–	–	26% (16/62)
Matsuoka [23]	1999	40	–	Holmium:YAG	80% (32/40)	–	5% (2/40)	15% (6/40)
Tawfiek [21]	1999	29	6F, 7.5F, 9.8F	Intact, EHL, PL, holmium:YAG	97% (28/29)	–	0% (0/29)	3% (1/29)
Erhard [20]	1996	39	6.9F, 7.5F, 10.8F, 13F	EHL, holmium:YAG, pulsed-dye	99% (38/39)	–	–	3% (1/39)
Total	–	507	–	–	80% (406/507)	–	–	–

LOS, length of stay in hospital; EHL, electrohydraulic lithotripsy; USL, ultrasonic lithotripsy; PL, pneumatic lithotripsy; YAG, yttrium-aluminum-garnet.

series, urine leaks were the most common postoperative complication [41,42]. Other authors have also reported successful laparoscopic ureterolithotomy for proximal ureteral calculi [43,44]. Although the laparoscopic approach to proximal ureteral stones is feasible, the procedure is currently indicated for stones when other endoscopic treatments have failed.

Open Surgery

Ureterolithotomy is reserved as salvage therapy for calculi when endourologic treatment has failed [1,40,45]. Open surgery results in essentially a 100% stone-free rate [40,45]. Liong and coworkers compared the choice of surgical incision (flank vs. dorsal lumbotomy) on postoperative recovery. Although both approaches were 100% successful, the flank incision was associated with a twofold higher complication rate (34% vs. 17%), longer hospitalization, and greater analgesic use [40].

Comparison of Treatments

Park and coworkers retrospectively compared URS with in situ SWL on a Dornier MPL9000 for proximal ureteral calculi [26]. In their 2-year experience, 301 patients were treated with SWL and 12 patients were treated with URS. Stone-free rates after a single session were 75% for URS and 72% for in situ SWL. For stones <1.0 cm, stone-free rates for SWL were 84% (182 of 216 patients); for stones >1.0 cm, only 42% of patients were rendered stone free. The combined URS stone-free rate was 88% for all stones, regardless of size.

Strohmaier and associates prospectively compared URS with SWL for treatment of proximal ureteral calculi [18]. In this study, the patients selected the primary and, if necessary, the secondary treatment. The stone-free rate for primary SWL was 76% (29/38), whereas primary URS was successful for the single patient selecting this treatment. Stones successfully treated with SWL had a mean diameter of 6.8 mm, whereas those for which SWL failed had a mean diameter of 9.4 mm. All patients for whom SWL failed selected secondary treatment with URS, and this secondary procedure was associated with an overall 97% stone-free rate.

Kupeli and colleagues compared URS with in situ SWL on a Siemens Lithostar [17]. Stone-free rates were not stratified by stone size; however, the mean stone diameter was 8 mm for stones treated with either URS or SWL. The stone-free rate for proximal ureteral calculi was 61%, and the stone-free rate for URS was 60%. The complication rate was significantly higher for URS (6 of 15 patients, 40%) than for SWL (18 of 458 patients, 3.9%). On the basis of complication rates alone, SWL was recommended as first-line treatment for proximal ureteral stones <1.0 cm in diameter.

Grasso and colleagues compared the efficacy of URS (27 patients; mean stone diameter, 9.9 mm) with SWL on a Siemens Lithostar (27 patients; mean stone diameter, 10.2 mm) for large proximal stones [14]. Stone-free rates of 62% and

97% were achieved with SWL and URS, respectively. Retreatment and auxiliary treatment were significantly higher in the SWL group than in the URS group (37% vs. 3.7%). In addition, treatment costs were higher and postoperative visits were more common in the SWL group. Grasso and associates also retrospectively evaluated 121 patients with renal or ureteral calculi for whom primary SWL treatment had failed. They concluded that SWL failures were more common among patients with large stones, hard stones, and those associated with urinary obstruction [46].

Maheshwari and associates compared PCNL with URS for large (>1.5 cm) impacted proximal stones for which SWL had failed [47]. A 100% immediate stone-free rate was noted for PCNL, as compared with a 55% rate for URS. At 3 months, however, the URS stone-free rate reached 85%. There were no intra-operative complications in either group, but two PCNL patients (8.7%) required blood transfusions.

Treatment Recommendations

The American Urological Association (AUA) has developed treatment guide-lines for ureteral stones above (proximal) or below (distal) the iliac vessels [1]. In the AUA guidelines, SWL is recommended as first-line therapy for most stones <1.0 cm above the iliac vessels. Placement of a ureteral stent to facilitate stone fragment passage after SWL did not effectively increase stone-free rates. For stones >1.0 cm above the iliac vessels, the guidelines recommended SWL, PCNL, or URS. However, a suggestion was made that URS was less effective for large stones. In our analysis, URS appears to be more advantageous for stones 1.0 to 1.5 cm in diameter. Many stones >1.5 cm are best treated with PCNL, but URS is still a reasonable option. PCNL is also effective salvage therapy if SWL and URS fail. The rare calculus refractory to endourological techniques is effectively managed with open or laparoscopic ureterolithotomy.

Management of Middle Ureteral Stones

Shock-Wave Lithotripsy

SWL treatment of middle ureteral calculi must take into account the anterior location of the ureter and the underlying pelvic bone [48,49]. Introduction of the Stryker frame modification for the gantry of the Dornier HM3 lithotripter enabled treatment of middle ureteral stones in the prone position, thereby avoiding attenuation of shock waves by the pelvic bones [50,51]. Jenkins and Gillenwater used the Stryker modification to treat 10 patients, achieving a 100% stone-free rate after a single treatment. To aid treatment, however, the authors also placed ureteral catheters by the stone in 9 of 10 cases [50]. With the use of the Stryker modifications, stone-free and retreatment rates with the Dornier HM3 since 1991 are 68%–100% and 0%–18%, respectively [4,48–50].

Cass reported on 53 patients with stones overlying the pelvic bone treated on the Dornier HM3 without the Stryker modification [52]. In this report, 33 patients with solitary middle ureteral stones had a stone-free rate of 75%, whereas 20 patients with multiple middle ureteral stones had a stone-free rate of 53%. All patients were treated in the prone position, and the majority of patients had a ureteral catheter placed to aid stone localization [52]. Placement of ureteral catheters prior to SWL for middle ureteral stones is controversial; no prospective, randomized studies have investigated the effect of stent placement on the treatment of middle ureteral stones by SWL with the Dornier HM3. Nakada and associates retrospectively reviewed 33 patients who underwent SWL on a Dornier HM3, with or without stent bypass. The overall stone-free rate for SWL was 73%. The stone-free rates for patients treated with stent bypass, pretreatment PCNL, and in situ were 71%, 75%, and 63%, respectively. For stones $\geq$10 mm in diameter, the stone-free rates after one treatment for stent bypass, pretreatment PCNL, and in situ treatment were 33%, 67%, and 33%, respectively. For stones <10mm in diameter, the success rates for the stent bypass, pretreatment PCNL, and in situ treatment groups were 82%, 100%, and 80%, respectively [53].

Second- and third-generation lithotripters have been associated with 51%–92% stone-free rates since 1994 (Table 3) [15–19,26,52,54]. Patient positioning is easier with higher-generation machines, and stone targeting is less cumbersome than with the Dornier HM3 lithotripter. Nonetheless, ureteral stents were used to facilitate stone targeting in 22% of patients in recent series [15–19,54]. Cass compared in situ SWL with bypass SWL on a Medstone STS lithotripter. The stone-free rates were 81% for patients with stents (n = 90) versus 60% for patients without stents (n = 10), although the difference was not statistically significant [55]. A prospective stent versus in situ study is also needed for treatment of middle ureteral stones with higher-generation lithotripters.

Ureteroscopy

New endoscopic technology has also benefited the treatment of middle ureteral stones. The newer semirigid ureteroscopes have been used predominantly for treatment of middle ureteral calculi, yielding stone-free rates of 89%–100% with no significant complications and no reported difficulty in accessing the middle ureter [22–27]. Using a combination of semirigid or flexible ureteroscopes, other studies have reported similar results with success rates of 93%–100% and no significant morbidity or access difficulty [16,20,21,55]. Of the intracorporeal lithotrites, the Ho:YAG laser is currently preferred [23–25,33]. Pneumatic lithotripsy in conjunction with semirigid ureteroscopy represents another effective lithotrite for middle ureteral calculi and may be a more cost-effective option [56–58]. In reports published since 1993, overall stone-free and retreatment rates for URS of middle ureteral stones were 75%–100% and 0%–12%, respectively (Table 4) [16–18,20–27,30,33,35,54].

TABLE 3. Results of shock-wave lithotripsy for middle ureteral calculi using the Dornier HM3 or higher-generation lithotripters

Author	Year	Lithotripter	Patients (stones)	Stone-free rate	ReTx	Aux proc.	Ureteral catheter	LOS (days)	Complications
Tiselius [9]	1991	Dornier HM3	62	97% (59/61)	34% (21/61)	–	98% (60/61)	–	–
Cass[a] [52]	1994	Dornier HM3	33	75% (18/24)	6% (2/33)	13% (3/24)	91% (30/33)	–	–
Cass[b] [52]	1994	Dornier HM3	20	53% (9/17)	5% (1/20)	24% (4/17)	95% (19/20)	–	–
Nakada [53]	1995	Dornier HM3	33	73% (19/26)	4%	19%	54% (14/26)	–	–
Subtotal	–	Dornier HM3	148	83% (105/128)	–	–	88% (123/140)	–	–
Cass [52]	1994	Medstone STS	101	80% (63/79)	6% (6/101)	8% (6/79)	–	–	–
Mobley [15]	1994	Lithostar	3077	83% (1733/2086)	12.2%	7%	25% (769/3077)	–	–
Grasso [16]	1995	Lithostar	4	75% (3/4)	0% (0/4)	25% (1/4)	0%	–	–
Bierkens [54]	1998	Lithostar	19	90% (17/19)	53% (10/19)	10.5% (2/19)	0%	1.1	15.7% (3/19)
Park [26]	1998	MPL9000	131	92% (120/131)	11% (15/131)	–	0%	–	–
Kupeli [17]	1998	Lithostar	396	51% (204/396)	–	–	0%	–	3.5% (14/396)
Gnanapragasam [19]	1999	MFL5000	35 (36)	89% (31/36)	–	11% (4/36)	0%	Outpatient	0% (0/36)
Strohmaier [18]	1999	Modulith, Compact	22	77% (17/22)	–	23% (5/22)	41% (9/22)	–	–
Subtotal	–	2nd and 3rd generation	3785	79% (2188/2773)	–	–	22% (778/3554)	–	–

[a] Includes only patients with single stones.
[b] Includes only patients with multiple stones.

TABLE 4. Treatment of middle ureteral stones with ureteroscopy

Author	Year	Patients	Size of ureteroscope	Modality of stone removal	Stone-free rate	LOS (days)	Complications	2nd procedure
Benrizi [35]	1993	11	6.5F, 7.5F	Pulsed-dye, Alexandrite laser	91% (10/11)	–	9% (1/11)	–
Grasso [16]	1995	15	6.9F, 7.5F	Pulsed-dye, EHL	93% (14/15)	–	–	7% (1/15)
Erhard [20]	1996	41	6.9F, 7.5F, 10.8F, 13F	EHL, holmium:YAG, pulsed-dye	90% (37/41)	Outpatient	–	10% (4/41)
Yiu [33]	1996	6	7F	Holmium:YAG	100% (6/6)	–	0% (0/6)	–
Bierkens [54]	1998	25	7.1F, 7.2F	Pulsed-dye	96% (24/25)	3.0	4% (1/25)	12% (3/25)
Kupeli [17]	1998	39	9.5F, 12F	EHL, USL, PL	77% (30/39)	–	26% (10/39)	–
Yip [27]	1998	17	8.5F, 9.5F	Holmium:YAG	100% (17/17)	–	–	–
Park [26]	1998	37	7.9F–11.5F	Intact or lithoclast	95% (35/37)	–	–	–
Pearle [25]	1998	16	6.9–8.5F	Alexandrite laser	75% (12/16)	–	–	–
Jung [30]	1998	36	6.5F	Alexandrite laser	86% (31/36)	–	3% (1/36)	6% (2/36)
Devarajan [24]	1998	53	7.5F	Holmium:YAG, Lithoclast	92% (49/53)	–	–	6% (3/53)
Strohmaier [18]	1999	8	7.5F–9.5F	Intact, EHL	75% (6/8)	–	–	–
Puppo [22]	1999	96	7F, 7.7F, 8F	EHL, PL	100% (96/96)	Outpatient	–	15% (14/96)
Tawfiek [21]	1999	19	6F, 7.5F, 9.8F	Intact, EHL, PL, holmium:YAG	100% (19/19)	Outpatient	0% (0/19)	0% (0/19)
Matsuoka [23]	1999	18	–	Holmium:YAG	89% (16/18)	–	0% (0/18)	6% (1/18)
Total	–	437	–	–	92% (402/437)	–	–	–

Percutaneous Surgery

PCNL is reserved for salvage therapy when URS and SWL fail. PCNL of middle stones was associated with a 58%–96% stone-free rate [37–40]. In the report by Clayman and colleagues, an overall complication rate of 65% was noted for PCNL of middle ureteral calculi [38]. PCNL of middle ureteral stones is feasible and effective, although the procedure is much more difficult than URS or SWL.

Laparoscopy

Transperitoneal and retroperitoneal laparoscopic ureterolithotomy have been used to successfully remove middle ureteral stones [41–44]. The laparoscopic approach is similar to that used for proximal stones. This treatment modality is recommended only in the event that SWL and URS fail.

Open Surgery

In the current era of endourology, an open approach to middle ureteral stones is exceedingly rare and is reserved for endourologic failures [59,60].

Comparison of Standard Treatment for Middle Ureteral Stones

The preferred approach for middle ureteral calculi (URS vs. SWL) is controversial. Advances in the flexible ureteroscope and downsizing of the flexible and semirigid ureteroscope have facilitated access to middle ureteral stones. Retrospective series have compared URS and SWL for treatment of middle ureteral stones. Kupeli and colleagues compared URS ($n = 39$) to in situ SWL ($n = 396$) on a Siemens Lithostar [17]. The overall mean stone diameter was 8 mm for patients treated with SWL or URS. For middle ureteral calculi, URS was associated with a 77% stone-free rate versus a 51% rate with SWL.

Bierkens and coworkers compared URS with pulsed-dye lithotripsy to in situ SWL on a Siemens Lithostar [54]. Although the ultimate success rates were comparable for SWL (90%) and URS (96%), the interval to becoming stone-free was <2 days for URS but up to 4 months for SWL. Also, 26% of patients (5/19) with residual fragments after SWL were rehospitalized for fever and required nephrostomy tube placement or antibiotics. The retreatment rate was 53% for SWL versus 12% for URS. Stone-free rates were not stratified by size: the mean stone size was 63 mm^2 for SWL and 50 mm^2 for URS. The authors reported that SWL was best for stones <50 mm^2 in size.

Park and coworkers compared URS with in situ SWL on a Dornier MPL9000 for middle ureteral calculi over a 2-year period [26]. Stone-free rates after a single session were 95% for URS and 70% for in situ SWL. For stones <1.0 cm, the stone-free rate for SWL was 78% (7 of 9 patients), and failed SWL in the single patient with a stone >1.0 cm. The combined stone-free rates in patients treated for ureteral stones with URS in all locations were unaffected by stone size.

Strohmaier and associates prospectively compared URS with SWL (Modulith or Compact lithotripter) in 30 patients with middle ureteral stones in whom the primary treatment was selected by the patient [18]. The stone-free rate was 77% (17 of 22 patients) for SWL and 75% (6 of 8 patients) for URS. The mean diameter of stones successfully treated with SWL was 8.1 mm; however, the mean diameter of stones successfully treated with URS was 14.3 mm. Among SWL patients, 41% had a stent placed prior to treatment. The success rate for the group receiving stents ($n = 9$) was 89%, compared with 69% for the group not receiving stents ($n = 13$) (no statistical comparison).

Grasso and colleagues compared URS with in situ SWL on a Lithostar-Plus for 19 patients with middle ureteral stones [16]. The stone-free rate for 15 patients (mean stone diameter, 7.6 mm) treated by URS was 93%, whereas the stone-free rate for 4 patients (mean stone diameter, 10.3 mm) treated with URS was 75%. In the study, SWL was associated with significantly higher retreatment and auxiliary treatment rates, more postoperative visits, and higher overall treatment costs.

Treatment Recommendations

Both URS and SWL are effective treatments for stones overlying the bony pelvis. To date, the superiority of one modality over the other has not been firmly established. For stones <1.0 cm in diameter, recent reports support treatment with in situ SWL [16,18,26,54]. In selecting this least invasive option, patients must accept a longer time to become stone-free and a higher likelihood of secondary procedures. The effect of stent placement on SWL efficiency will require completion of a prospective, randomized trial. However, if stent placement is indicated, URS is a short step away and may be the most definitive treatment. Based on the report by Strohmaier and colleagues, stones >1.0 cm in diameter may best be treated with URS [18]. A paucity of results stratified by stone size and stone location limits recommendations for treatment based on stone size [17,20,21,33,54]. However, PCNL is used predominantly for salvage therapy if URS fails. In rare instances, a large-diameter middle ureteral stone warrants first-line treatment with PCNL. Laparoscopic or open stone removal is recommended only as salvage treatment.

Management of Distal Ureteral Stones

Optimal management of distal ureteral stones is one of the more hotly debated topics in endourology. Both URS and SWL are highly effective. Furthermore, in some instances, short-term placement of a ureteral stent results in spontaneous stone passage. Leventhal and associates prospectively evaluated spontaneous stone passage in 17 patients whose disease was initially managed with a ureteral stent [61]. After stent removal approximately 2 weeks later, 83% of patients spontaneously passed their stones after an average of 5.5 days (range, 0–25 days). The three patients for whom treatment by stent placement failed were treated with URS.

Shock-Wave Lithotripsy

The stone-free rates for patients with distal ureteral calculi are 77%–100% for those treated by use of the Dornier HM3 [4,49,62–65] and 59%-97% for those treated with second- and third-generation lithotripters [11,12,14–19,62,63,64–67] (Table 5). The advantage of stent placement prior to SWL has not been clearly shown. Indeed, Marberger and colleagues reported a 95% stone-free rate for 161 distal stones treated with in situ SWL on a Siemens Lithostar [68].

Ureteroscopy

For series published since 1996, the contemporary stone-free rates for URS using smaller-caliber ureteroscopes and improved lithotrites are 86%–100% (Table 6) [17,18,21–24,26,27,30,54,63,64–67,72]. These results are similar to the success rates of 83%–94% reported for older series [69–71]. However, with current instrumentation the incidence of ureteral perforation is less than 4% [26,30,64,66,72], and the incidence of strictures is less than 2% [26,66,72].

Laparoscopy

Anecdotal reports have described laparoscopic ureterolithotomy. Both Micali and coworkers and Raboy and colleagues successfully removed distal stones using a transperitoneal approach [43,73]. Failed endourologic techniques prompted laparoscopy in the majority of cases, although one cystinuric patient in whom URS and dissolution therapy failed was treated primarily.

Open Surgery

Ureterolithotomy is predominantly a rare salvage procedure for endourologic failures. In a report by Kane and coworkers, eight patients underwent ureterolithotomy for failed endoscopic procedures (three patients), impacted stones (two patients), simultaneous anatrophic nephrolithotomy (two patients), or simultaneous prostatectomy (one patient) [59]. Recently, Paik and colleagues reported seven ureterolithotomies; the indications were failed endoscopy (five patients), ureteral stricture (one patient), and concurrent colon surgery (one patient). All stones were >2.0 cm in diameter [60].

Comparison of Standard Treatment for Distal Stones

The optimal treatment for distal ureteral stones is controversial. Numerous retrospective studies have compared URS and SWL. Turk and Jenkins recom-

TABLE 5. Results of shock-wave lithotripsy for distal ureteral calculi using Dornier HM3 or higher-generation lithotripters

Author	Year	Lithotripter	Patients	Stone-free rate	ReTx	Aux proc.	Ureteral catheter	LOS (days)	Complications
Anderson [62]	1994	Dornier HM3	27	96% (26/27)	3% (2/65)	6% (4/65)	0%	–	0% (0/27)
Erturk [65]	1993	Dornier HM3	312	81% (199/245)	4% (14/312)	–	79%	–	5% (16/312)
Tiselius [9]	1993	Dornier HM3	212	96.7% (205/212)	23% (49/212)	7% (15/212)	62%	–	–
Turk [63]	1999	Dornier HM3	44	78% (35/44)	–	–	–	–	–
Subtotal	–	Dornier HM3	595	88% (465/528)	–	–	–	3	5% (16/339)
Chang [12]	1993	Lithostar	32	59% (19/32)	0% (0/32)	41% (13/32)	0%	–	–
Voce [11]	1993	MPL9000	285	97% (276/285)	34% (95/285)	3% (9/285)	4%	Outpatient	0%
Anderson [62]	1994	Lithostar	22	84% (18/22)	14% (3/22)	14% (3/22)	18%	Outpatient	0% (0/27)
Mobley [15]	1994	Lithostar	7271	83% (4084/4921)	10%	9%	13%	–	–
Frabboni [14]	1994	MPL9000	285	97% (276/285)	17% (49/285)	4% (12/285)	4%	–	0% (0/285)
Grasso [16]	1995	Lithostar	11	64% (7/11)	0% (0/11)	18% (2/11)	–	–	–
Kupeli [17]	1998	Lithostar	726	42% (306/726)	–	–	–	–	5% (36/726)
Park [26]	1998	MPL9000	131	92% (120/131)	11% (15/131)	–	–	–	–
Eden [64]	1998	Modulith	313	75% single stones, 50% multiple stones	–	26% (81/313)	16%	Outpatient	4% (14/313)
Strohmaier [18]	1999	Modulith, Compact	37	59% (22/37)	–	41% (15/37)	16% (6/37)	–	–
Pardalidis [66]	1999	Lithostar	395	93% (368/395) 1 tx, 99% (391/395) 2 tx	6% (23/368)	1% (4/368)	–	Outpatient	4% (17/395)
Turk [63]	1999	HM3/MFL5000	91	73%	15% (14/91)	7% (6/91)	–	–	0% (0/91)
Peschel [67]	1999	MFL5000	40	90% (36/40)	0% (0/40)	10% (4/40)	–	–	0% (0/40)
Gnanapragasam [19]	1999	MFL5000	62	86% (53/62)	–	15% (9/62)	8%	Outpatient	0% (0/62)
Subtotal	–	2nd and 3rd generation	9701	78% (5519/7038)	–	–	–	–	4% (37/1045)

TABLE 6. Treatment of distal ureteral stones with URS

Author	Year	Patients (stones)	Size of ureteroscope	Modality of stone removal	Stone-free rate	LOS (days)	Complications	2nd procedure
Jung [30]	1996	156	6.5F	Alexandrite laser	94.5% (148/156)	–	0% (0/156)	5% (8/156)
Netto [72]	1997	322	11.5F	Basket	98.1% (316/322)	0.15	4.3% (14/322)	0% (0/322)
Kupeli [17]	1998	430	9.5F, 12F	EHL, USL, lithoclast	91.9% (395/430)	–	12.6% (54/430)	–
Bierkens [54]	1998	80	7.2F	Pulsed dye	99% (79/80)	3.2	0% (0/80)	7% (6/80)
Eden [64]	1998	134	7F, 9.5F, 11.5F	Lithoclast	89.5% (120/134)	1.1	2.2% (3/134)	6.0% (8/134)
Park [26]	1998	66	7.9F–11.5F	Intact or lithoclast	86.4% (57/66)	–	–	–
Pearle [25]	1998	48	6.9–8.5F	Alexandrite laser	94% (45/48)	–	–	–
Devarajan [24]	1998	102	7.5F	Holmium:YAG	93% (95/102)	–	–	2% (2/102)
Peschel [67]	1999	40	6.5F, 9.5F	Intact, lithoclast	100% (40/40)	–	0% (0/40)	0% (0/40)
Tawfiek [21]	1999	34	6F, 7.5F, 9.8F	Intact, EHL, PL, holmium:YAG	100% (34/34)	Outpatient	0% (0/34)	0% (0/34)
Turk [63]	1999	96	7.5–9.5F	Intact, pulsed dye laser	95% (93/96)	–	5.2% (5/96)	3.1% (3/96)
Puppo [22]	1999	220	7F, 7.7F, 8F	EHL, PL	99.6% (219/220)	–	–	6.3% (14/220)
Strohmaier [18]	1999	40	7.5F–9.5F	Intact, EHL	97% (39/40)	–	–	–
Pardalidis [66]	1999	228[a] (238)	11.5F	USL, EHL[b]	92% (219/238)	1.3	2.5% (6/238)	4.2% (10/238)
Matsuoka [23]	1999	30	–	Holmium:YAG	93% (28/30)	–	3% (1/30)	0% (0/30)
Pearle [unpublished, 2000]	2000	32	6.9F, 11.5F	Intact, alexandrite or holmium:YAG laser, EHL	100% (29/29)	75% Outpatients	25% (8/32)	0% (0/32)
Total	–	2058	–	–	95% (1956/2055)	–	–	–

[a] Includes 3 patients in whom the stone was treated from a percutaneous antegrade approach.
[b] Includes 12 patients in whom SWL had previously failed.

mended URS for distal stones after reviewing their series of patients treated with a Dornier HM3 (44 patients) or Dornier MFL5000 (47 patients) versus URS (96 patients). Stone-free rates favored URS (95%) over SWL (83% for the HM3, 77% for the MFL5000), but complications occurred only with URS (5.2%). The mean stone diameters for patients successfully treated with URS, the Dornier HM3 lithotripter, and the MFL5000 were 9.8, 9.9, and 7.3 mm, respectively. The stones for which treatment with URS failed had a mean diameter of 14.3 mm, whereas stones for which treatment with the Dornier HM3 failed had a mean diameter of 12.3 mm [63].

Eden and associates noted a 90% stone-free rate for 134 patients treated with URS and 75% for 313 patients treated with in situ SWL on a Modulith SL [64]. Multiple stones were more effectively treated with URS (89% stone-free rate) than SWL (50% stone-free rate). Stones <8 mm in diameter were associated with a stone-free rate of 89%–100%, compared with 11%–75% for stones >8 mm in diameter. The stone-free rates for URS were not size-dependent. The authors recommended in situ SWL for single stones <8 mm.

Anderson and coworkers reported stone-free rates of 96% for the Dornier HM3 SWL, 84% for Lithostar SWL, and 100% for ureteroscopy [62]. The mean stone sizes for Dornier HM3 SWL, Lithostar SWL, and URS were 35, 24, and 30 mm^2, respectively. URS was associated with longer operation times, more common use of general anesthesia, prolonged convalescence, and routine stent placement. These investigators recommended SWL as first-line treatment and URS as a salvage therapy for SWL failures.

Several prospective randomized trials have also compared SWL and URS treatment of distal ureteral calculi. Peschel and colleagues noted 100% URS stone-free rates ($n = 40$) and 90% SWL stone-free rates with a Dornier MFL5000 ($n = 40$) [66]. For stones <5 mm and >5 mm in diameter, the SWL stone-free rates were 85% and 95%, respectively. No complications were noted in either group, but operative time favored URS. Patient satisfaction was 100% for URS and 85% for SWL. Based on these results, URS was the recommended first-line distal stone treatment.

On the other hand, Pearle and colleagues prospectively randomized 32 patients with distal stones (diameter <15 mm) to URS or SWL with a Dornier HM3 [unpublished, MS Pearle, 2001]. A 100% stone-free rate was noted for both treatments, but SWL patients had significantly shorter operative times. In addition, SWL was associated with less postoperative discomfort, fewer complications, and greater patient satisfaction, although the differences were not statistically significant. For distal stones <15 mm, either treatment is acceptable, although Pearle and associates recommended SWL using a Dornier HM3 as first-line treatment because it is less invasive.

Treatment Recommendations

Treatment is influenced by many factors. However, patient preference plays an important role with distal stones. The AUA guidelines recommend definitive treatment with either URS or SWL. The guidelines do not support stent place-ment to improve SWL stone-free rates. Because high success rates have been achieved with both SWL and URS, optimal first-line therapy for distal stones is controversial, and either treatment modality is acceptable.

Conclusions

With the success of endourologic treatment of ureteral calculi, most ureteral calculi are successfully managed with either SWL or URS. The coexistence of two effective modalities for treatment of ureteral calculi has created controversy. The battle for optimal treatment of ureteral calculi has been amplified with the increas-ing use of URS secondary to improvements in ureteroscope design and instru-mentation. Patient preference, physician familiarity, and instrument availability are other factors that may influence treatment. Only prospective, randomized trials employing state-of-the-art technology will determine the optimal treatment algorithms for ureteral calculi and help resolve management controversies.

References

1. Segura JW, Preminger GM, Assimos DG, Dretler SP, Lingeman JE, Macaluso JN Jr (1997) Ureteral stones clinical guidelines panel summary report on the management of ureteral calculi. J Urol 158:1915–1921
2. Ueno A, Kawamura T, Ogawa A, Takayasu H (1977) Relation of spontaneous passage of calculi to size. Urology 10:544–546
3. Mueller SC, Wilbert D, Thueroff JW, Alken P (1986) Extracorporeal shock wave lithotripsy of ureteral stones: clinical experience and experimental findings. J Urol 135:831–834
4. Manzone DJ, Chiang B (1988) Extracorporeal shock wave lithotripsy of stones in the upper, mid and lower ureter. J Endourol 2:107–111
5. Liong ML, Clayman RV, Gittes RF, Lingeman JE, Lyon ES (1989) Treatment options for proximal ureteral urolithiasis. J Urol 141:504–509
6. El-Gammal MY, Fouda AA, Meshef AW, Abu-Elk-Magd AM, Farag FA, El-Katib SE (1992) Management of ureteral stones by extracorporeal shock wave lithotripsy using Lithostar lithotriptor. J Urol 148:1086–1087
7. Danuser H, Ackermann DK, Marth DC, Studer UE, Zingg E (1993) Extracorporeal shock wave lithotripsy in situ or after push-up for upper ureteral calculi: a prospec-tive randomized trial. J Urol 150:824–826
8. Albala DM, Clayman RV, Meretyk S (1991) Extracorporeal shock wave lithotripsy for proximal ureteral calculi: to stint or not to stint? J Endourol 5:277–281
9. Tiselius H (1991) Anesthesia-free in situ extracorporeal shockwave lithotripsy of ureteral stones. J Urol 146:8–12
10. Cass AS (1992) Do upper ureteral stones need to be manipulated (pushback) into the kidney before extracorporeal shock lithotrispy? J Urol 147:349–351
11. Voce S, Dal Pozzo C, Arnone S, Montanari F (1993) "In situ" echo-guided extracor-poreal shock wave lithotripsy of ureteral stones. Methods and results with Dornier MPL 9000. Scand J Urol Nephrol 27:469–473

12. Chang SC, Kuo HC, Hsu T (1993) Extracorporeal shock wave lithotripsy for obstructed proximal ureteral stones. Eur Urol 24:177–184
13. Ilker NY, Alican Y, Simsek F, Turkeri LN, Akdas A (1994) Ureteral extracorporeal shock wave lithotripsy using Dornier MFL 5000. J Endourol 8:13–15
14. Frabboni R, Santi V, Ronchi M, Gaiani S, Costanza N, Ferrari G, Ferrari P, Corrado G, Concetti S, Fornarola V (1994) In situ echoguided extracorporeal shock wave lithotripsy of ureteric stones with the Dornier MPL 9000: a multicentric study group. Br J Urol 73:487–493
15. Mobley TB, Myers DA, McK. Jenkins J, Grine WB, Jordan WR (1994) Effects of stents on lithotripsy of ureteral calculi: treatment results with 18825 calculi using the lithostar lithotriptor. J Urol 152:53–56
16. Grasso M, Beaghler M, Loisides P (1995) The case for primary endoscopic management of upper urinary tract calculi: cost and outcome assessment of 112 primary ureteral calculi. Urology 45:372–376
17. Kupeli B, Biri H, Isen K, Onaran M, Alkibay T, Karaoglan U, Bozkirli I (1998) Treatment of ureteral stones: comparison of extracorporeal shock wave lithotripsy and endourologic alternatives. Eur Urol 34:474–479
18. Strohmaier WL, Schubert G, Rosenkranz T, Weigl A (1999) Comparison of extracorporeal shock wave lithotripsy and ureteroscopy in the treatment of ureteral calculi: a prospective study. Eur Urol 36:376–379
19. Gnanapragasam VJ, Ramsden PDR, Murthy LSN, Thomas DJ (1999) Primary in situ extracorporeal shock wave lithotripsy in the management of ureteric calculi: results with a third-generation lithotripter. BJU Int 84:770–774
20. Erhard M, Salwen J, Bagley DH (1996) Ureteroscopic removal of mid and proximal ureteral calculi. J Urol 155:38–42
21. Tawfiek ER, Bagley DH (1999) Management of upper urinary tract calculi with ureteroscopic techniques. Urology 53:25–31
22. Puppo P, Ricciotti G, Bozzo W, Introini C (1999) Primary endoscopic treatment of ureteric calculi. Eur Urol 36:48–52
23. Matsuoka K, Iida S, Inoue M, Yoshii S, Arai K, Tomiyasu K, Noda S (1999) Endoscopic lithotrispy with the holmium:YAG laser. Lasers Surg Med 25:389–395
24. Devarajan R, Ashraf M, Beck RO, Lemberger RJ, Taylor MC (1998) Holmium: YAG lasertripsy for ureteric calculi: an experience of 300 procedures. Br J Urol 82: 342–347
25. Pearle MS, Sech SM, Cobb CG, Riley JR, Clark PJ, Preminger GM, Drach GW, Roehrborn CG (1998) Safety and efficacy of the alexandrite laser for the treatment of renal and ureteral calculi. Urology 51:33–38
26. Park H, Park M, Park T (1998) Two-year experience with ureteral stones: extracorporeal shockwave lithotripsy v ureteroscopic manipulation. J Endourol 12:501–504
27. Yip KH, Lee CW, Tam PC (1998) Holmium laser lithotripsy for ureteral calculi: an outpatient procedure. J Endourol 12:241–246
28. Harmon WJ, Sershon PD, Blute ML, Patterson DE, Segura JW (1997) Ureteroscopy: current practice and long-term complications. J Urol 157:28–32
29. Yang SSD, Hong JS (1996) Electrohydraulic lithotripsy of upper ureteral calculi with semirigid ureteroscope. J Endourol 10:27–29
30. Jung P, Wolff JM, Mattelaer P, Jakse G (1996) Role of lasertripsy in the management of ureteral calculi: experience with alexandrite laser system in 232 patients. J Endourol 10:345–348

31. Elashry OM, Elbahnasy AM, Rao GS, Nakada SY, Clayman RV (1997) Flexible ureteroscopy: Washington University experience with the 9.3F and 7.5F flexible ureteroscopes. J Urol 157:2074–2080

32. Teichman JMH, Vassar GJ, Bishoff JT, Bellman GC (1998) Holmium:YAG lithotripsy yields smaller fragments than lithoclast, pulsed dye laser or electrohydraulic lithotripsy. J Urol 159:17–23

33. Yiu MK, Liu PL, Yiu TF, Chan AYT (1996) Clinical experience with holmium:YAG laser lithotripsy of ureteral calculi. Lasers Surg Med 19:103–106

34. Elashry OM, DiMeglio RB, Nakada SY, McDougall EM, Clayman RV (1996) Intra-corporeal electrohydraulic lithotripsy of ureteral and renal calculi using small caliber (1.9F) electrohydraulic lithotripsy probes. J Urol 156:1581–1585

35. Benizri E, Wodey J, Amiel J, Toubol J (1993) Comparison of 2 pulsed lasers for lithotripsy of ureteral calculi: report on 154 patients. J Urol 150:1803–1805

36. Francesca F, Scattoni V, Nava L, Pompa P, Grasso M, Rigatti P (1995) Failures and complications of transurethral ureteroscopy in 297 cases: conventional rigid instruments vs. small caliber semirigid ureteroscopes. Eur Urol 28:112–115

37. Segura JW, Patterson DE, LeRoy AJ (1985) Percutaneous removal of kidney stones: review of 1000 cases. J Urol 134:1077–1081

38. Clayman RV, Surya V, Miller RP (1984) Percutaneous nephrolithotomy: extraction of renal and ureteral calculi from 100 patients. J Urol 131:868

39. Reddy PK, Hulbert JC, Lange PH (1985) Percutaneous removal of renal and ureteral calculi: experience with 400 cases. J Urol 134:662–665

40. Liong M, Clayman R, Gittes R (1989) Treatment options for proximal ureteral urolithiasis: review and recommendations. J Urol 141:504

41. Gaur DD (1993) Retroperitoneal laparoscopic ureterolithotomy: our experience in 12 patients. J Endourol 7:501–503

42. Harewood LM, Webb DR, Pope AJ (1994) Laparoscopic ureterolithotomy: the results of an initial series, and an evaluation of its role in the management of ureteric calculi. Br J Urol 74:170–176

43. Micali S, Moore RG, Averch TD, Adams JB, Kavoussi LR (1997) The role of laparoscopy in the treatment of renal and ureteral calculi. J Urol 157:463–466

44. Bellman GC, Smith AD (1994) Special considerations in the technique of laparoscopic ureterolithotomy. J Urol 151:146–149

45. Netto NR Jr, De Almeida Claro JF, Ferreira U, Lemos GC (1991) Lumbar ureteric stones: which is the best treatment? Urology 38:443–446

46. Grasso M, Loisides P, Beaghler M, Bagley D (1995) The case for primary endoscopic management of upper urinary tract calculi: I A critical review of 121 extracorporeal shock-wave lithotripsy failures. Urology 45:363–371

47. Maheshwari PN, Oswal AT, Andankar M, Nanjappa KM, Bansal M (1999) Is antegrade ureteroscopy better than retrograde ureteroscopy for impacted large upper ureteral calculi? J Endourol 13:441–444

48. Fetner CD, Preminger GM, Seger J, Lea LA (1988) Treatment of ureteral calculi by extracorporeal shock wave lithotripsy at a multi-use center. J Urol 139:1192–1194

49. Miller K, Bachor R, Hautmann R (1988) Extracorporeal shock wave lithotripsy in the prone position: technique, indications, results. J Endourol 2:113–115

50. Jenkins AD, Gillenwater JY (1988) Extracorporeal shock wave lithotripsy in the prone position: treatment of stones in the distal ureter of anomalous kidney. J Urol 139:911–915

51. Leveilee RJ, Zabbo A, Barrette D (1994) Stryker frame adaptation of the HM3 lithotriptor for treatment of distal ureteral calculi. J Urol 151:391–393
52. Cass AS (1994) Extracorporeal shock-wave lithotrispy for stones in middle third of ureter (overlying pelvic bone). Urology 43:182–186
53. Nakada SY, Pearle MS, Soble JJ, Gardner SM, McClennan BL, Clayman RV (1995) Extracorporeal shock-wave lithotripsy of middle ureteral stones: are ureteral stents necessary? Urology 46:649–652
54. Bierkens AF, Hendrikx AJM, De La Rosette JJ, Stultiens GNM, Beerlage HP, Arends AJ, Debruyne FMJ (1998) Treatment of mid and lower ureteric calculi: extracorporeal shock-wave lithotripsy vs laser ureteroscopy. A comparison of costs, morbidity, and effectiveness. Br J Urol 81:31–35
55. Cass AS (1993) Nonstent or noncatheter extracorporeal shock-wave lithotripsy for ureteral stones. Urology 43:178–181
56. Knispel HH, Klan R, Heicappell R, Miller K (1998) Pneumatic lithotripsy applied through deflected working channel of miniureteroscope: results in 143 patients. J Endourol 12:513–515
57. Kok TP, Ming TS, Consigliere D (1998) Ureteroscopic lithoclast lithotripsy: a cost-effective option. J Endourol 12:341–344
58. Huang S, Patel H, Bellman GC (1998) Cost effectiveness of electrohydraulic lithotripsy v candela pulsed-dye laser in management of the distal ureteral stone. J Endourol 12:237–239
59. Kane CJ, Bolton DM, Stoller ML (1995) Current indications for open stone surgery in an endourology center. Urology 45:218–221
60. Paik ML, Wainstein MA, Spirnak JP, Hampel N, Resnick MI (1998) Current indications for open stone surgery in the treatment of renal and ureteral calculi. J Urol 159:374–378
61. Leventhal EK, Rozanski TA, Crain TW, Deshon GE Jr (1995) Indwelling ureteral stents as definitive therapy for distal ureteral calculi. J Urol 153:34–36
62. Anderson KR, Keetch DW, Albala DM, Chandhoke PS, McClennan BL, Clayman RV (1994) Optimal therapy for the distal ureteral stone: extracorporeal shock wave lithotripsy versus ureteroscopy. J Urol 152:62–65
63. Turk TM, Jenkins AD (1999) A comparison of ureteroscopy to in situ extracorporeal shock wave lithotripsy for the treatment of distal ureteral calculi. J Urol 161:45–46
64. Eden CG, Mark IR, Gupta RR, Eastman J, Shrotri NC, Tiptaft RC (1998) Intracorporeal or extracorporeal lithotripsy for distal ureteral calculi? Effect of stone size and multiplicity on success rate. J Endourol 12:307
65. Erturk E, Herrman E, Cockett AT (1993) Extracorporeal shock wave lithotripsy for distal ureteral stones. J Urol 149:1425–1426
66. Pardalidis NP, Kosmaoglou EV, Kapotis CG (1999) Endoscopy vs. extracorporeal shockwave lithotripsy in the treatment of distal ureteral stones: ten years' experience. J Endourol 13:161–164
67. Peschel R, Janetschek G, Bartsch G (1999) Extracorporeal shock wave lithotripsy versus ureteroscopy for distal ureteral calculi: a prospective randomized study. J Urol 162:1909–1912
68. Marberger M, Hofbauer J, Turk C, Hobarth K, Albrecht W (1994) Management of ureteric stones. Eur Urol 25:265–272
69. Blute ML, Segura JW, Patterson DE (1988) Ureteroscopy. J Urol 139:510–512
70. Keating MA, Heney NM, Young HH II, Kerr WS Jr, O'Leary MP, Dretler SP (1986) Ureteroscopy: the initial experience. J Urol 135:689–693

71. Daniels GF Jr, Garnett JE, Carter MF (1988) Ureteroscopic results and complications: experience with 130 cases. J Urol 139:710–713
72. Netto NR Jr, De Almeida Claro J, Esteves SC, Andrade EFM (1997) Ureteroscopic stone removal in the distal ureter. Why change? J Urol 157:2081–2083
73. Raboy A, Ferzli GS, Ioffreda R, Albert PS (1992) Laparoscopic ureterolithotomy. Urology 39:223–225

Review of the Clinical Guidelines for Staghorn Calculi

Kikuo Nutahara[1], Eiji Higashihara[1], Akito Yamaguchi[2], and Mikio Kanemura[3]

Summary. Reviewing the clinical guidelines for staghorn calculi of the American Urological Association (AUA), European Association of Urology (EAU), and the literature appearing after their survey, guidelines for staghorn calculi are proposed for the Japanese Urological Association (JUA). A patient newly diagnosed with staghorn calculi needs to be fully informed about active treatment modalities, including their clinical efficacy and adverse events. Standard patients with staghorn calculi must be introduced to a specialist, because they will receive active treatment. Percutaneous nephrolithotomy (PNL), followed by extracorporeal shock-wave lithotripsy (ESWL) or repeat percutaneous procedure, should be recommended as the first-line treatment modality for standard patients with staghorn calculi. Open surgery is indicated for a limited number of patients.

Key Words. Staghorn calculi, Guidelines, PNL, ESWL, Open surgery

Natural History of Staghorn Calculi

Treatment of patients with staghorn calculi remains the most complex problem in modern urology. Although Libertino et al. [1] reported that medical therapy is the first-line treatment for asymptomatic, especially solitary, staghorn calculi, Rous and Turner claimed that avoiding surgery was the worst alternative and 30% of patients without operation died of renal failure and/or sepsis [2]. Koga et al. studied 61 patients with staghorn calculi treated conservatively; 7 of 61 patients (11.5%) died of uremia due to bilateral staghorn calculi. The morbidity and mortality rates following conservative treatment were higher than those

[1] Department of Urology, Kyorin University, School of Medicine, 6-20-2 Shinkawa, Mitaka, Tokyo 181-8611, Japan
[2] Department of Urology, Hara Sanshin Hospital, 1-8 Oohiro-cho, Hakata-ku, Fukuoka 812-0033, Japan
[3] Department of Urology, Kameda General Hospital, 1344 Higashimachi, Kamogawa, Chiba 296-0041, Japan

following surgical treatment by nephrectomy, extended pyelolithotomy, nephrolithotomy, or partial nephrectomy [3]. Teichman et al. reported that the overall rate of functional deterioration of the kidney for patients with staghorn calculi was 28% during 7.7 years of follow-up. Renal deterioration in patients with staghorn calculi was more frequently associated with solitary than with non-solitary kidneys, recurrent than nonrecurrent stones, and complete than partial staghorn calculi. No patient with complete clearance of fragments died of renal-related causes, compared with 3% of those without clearance of fragments and 67% of those who refused treatment ($P < 0.001$) [4]. If a struvite stone (infection stone) is not removed completely, the patient will continue to have urinary tract infections and the stone will begin to grow again. Therefore, to cure infection stones, they must be removed completely [5]. The American Urological Association (AUA) Nephrolithiasis Clinical Guidelines Panel recommended that a newly diagnosed struvite staghorn calculus should receive some active treatment rather than be followed with conservative observation. The panel recommended that percutaneous nephrolithotomy (PNL), followed by extracorporeal shock-wave lithotripsy (ESWL) or repeat PNL as necessary, should be selected as the first-line treatment for most patients with staghorn calculi [6,7].

Meta-analyses of the Data

The AUA clinical guidelines were basically a summary of the published treatments with statistical analyses of their outcome, as opposed to an implicit approach relying solely on expert opinion, without an open description of the evidence considered. The total number of articles reviewed was 1250 in the AUA clinical guidelines for staghorn calculi, and the last Medline search before data abstraction included all related manuscripts as of January 1993 [7]. New clinical guidelines on urolithiasis edited by the Japanese Urological Association (JUA) have been planned. Based on the AUA clinical guidelines for staghorn calculi and survey of the articles appearing after 1993, a chapter on staghorn calculi in the JUA guidelines is being developed. According to the opinions of specialists, journals that were not listed on Medline were also searched, for example, the Japanese Journal of Endourology and ESWL. Of the 74 new articles analyzed, 35 elicited abstracts and 30 were referenced. Excluding 2 papers related solely to epidemiology, 28 papers were included in addition to the 110 articles used in the AUA guidelines. These data were subjected to meta-analysis. The most important outcomes of various treatment modalities are summarized in Table 1. The stone-free rate seems to be highest with the combined treatment modalities of PNL and ESWL, although statistical comparison is not possible due to the different backgrounds of the papers. A prospective, randomized, controlled study by Meretyk and his associates revealed the advantages of a combined PNL and ESWL approach over ESWL monotherapy for the treatment of patients with staghorn calculi after the publication of the AUA clinical guidelines for staghorn calculi (Table 2) [8].

TABLE 1. Outcomes of various treatments for staghorn calculi[a]

Outcome	ESWL	PNL	PNL + ESWL	Open
Stone-free rate	1173/2275	458/593	800/961	2087/2555
	51.56%	77.23%	83.25%	81.68%
Acute complications	459/1232	58/1026	190/808	657/2373
	37.26%	5.65%	23.51%	27.69%
Long-term complications	3/54	12/93	No data	219/1549
	5.56%	12.90%		14.14%

ESWL, extracorporeal shock-wave lithotrupsy; PNL, percutaneous nephrolithotomy.
[a] Based on the literature adopted in the AUA guidelines for staghorn calculi, an additional 28 articles on the treatment of staghorn calculi were meta-analyzed.

TABLE 2. Treatment outcome[a]

Outcome	ESWL (27 patients)	PNL + ESWL (23 patients)
% stone-free rate (6 months)	6/27	17/23**
	22%	74%
Rate of septic complications	15/27	2/23**
	56%	9%
Rate of ancillary procedures	8/27	1/23*
	30%	4%
Mean total treatment length (months)	6	1**
Mean hospitalization days	16.8	13.7

* $P < 0.05$, ** $P < 0.01$, significant difference between two modalities.
[a] Meretyk et al. [8].

Proposal by an Ad Hoc Committee of the JUA

Definition and Quantification of Staghorn Calculi

Staghorn calculi are defined as stones that fill almost all calices and the renal pelvis. Although the term "partial staghorn calculi" is often used, there is no agreement on how this term should be defined. Winfield et al. reported that a partial staghorn stone was defined as one that filled the renal pelvis plus one or more calices [9]. The treatment recommendations and results reported for the treatment of staghorn calculi are highly variable. One of the reasons for such varied results is the difficulty of accurately assessing the stone burden in patients with staghorn calculi. Lam et al. reported that the stone burden was measured as the stone surface area, calculated by microcomputer. They suggested that the use of stone surface area allowed for meaningful comparisons among treatment results from different institutions and modalities [10]. Although stone surface area appears to be a highly accurate and reproducible method to assess the stone burden in patients with staghorn calculi, this method cannot be generalized due to its difficulty. In this guideline, staghorn calculi of apparently small stone burden are defined as "small volume staghorn calculi," and the guidelines apply this to the treatment of renal stones more than 2 cm in diameter. Although four treatment modalities are shown in Table 1—ESWL, PNL, combined treatment with PNL and ESWL, and open surgery—lithotripsy using ureteroscopy is included as an active stone-removing treatment modality in this guideline.

Standard Patient

A standard patient is defined as a newly diagnosed adult patient who has radio-opaque complete staghorn calculi, including struvite stones, who has an almost normally functioning affected kidney, and whose overall physical condition permits the performance of usual surgical procedures, including the use of anesthesia. Patients with staghorn calculi composed mainly of cystine and uric acid are excluded from the standard patient group. The recommended standards and guidelines apply to the treatment of standard patients, and the options apply to the other, nonstandard patients.

Summary

A newly diagnosed patient with staghorn calculi needs to be fully informed about the active treatment modalities, including their clinical efficacy and adverse events. Standard patients with staghorn calculi must be introduced to a specialist, because they will receive active treatment. Percutaneous nephrolithotomy, followed by ESWL or repeat percutaneous procedure, should be recommended as first-line treatment for standard patients with staghorn calculi. Open surgery is indicated for a limited number of patients.

Recommendations

There are three graded treatment recommendations as well as AUA clinical guidelines. A standard has the least flexibility among the three recommendations. An option is the most flexible recommendation.

Standard

1. A standard patient diagnosed with staghorn calculi needs to be fully informed about active stone-removing treatment modalities, that is PNL, ESWL, ureteroscopy, combined treatment with PNL and ESWL, and open surgery, including their clinical efficacy and adverse effects.

Guidelines

1. Active stone-removing treatment is desirable for newly diagnosed standard patients with staghorn calculi.

2. In a patient with a positive urinary tract infection, treatment with antibiotics should be performed before the active stone-removing procedure. There is no scientific article describing which antibiotics should be used and how long they

should be used. Based on expert opinion, antibiotic chemotherapy should be started before active stone removal, because severe urinary tract infection may induce urosepsis.

    3. PNL, followed by ESWL and/or repeat percutaneous stone removal as necessary, should be used for most patients with staghorn calculi [8,11,12].

    4. ESWL monotherapy is not indicated for standard patients with staghorn calculi as a first-line treatment [13].

    5. Open surgery is not indicated for standard patients with staghorn calculi as a first-line treatment [14].

Options

1. ESWL with double J stenting, PNL monotherapy, and lithotripsy using ureteroscopy are indicated for patients with small-volume staghorn calculi [11,12,15–19].
2. Open surgery is indicated when the treatment of staghorn calculi, using ESWL, PNL, and ureteroscopy appropriately, will fail [20].
3. Nephrectomy is considered a reasonable treatment alternative for patients with a poorly functioning kidney.
4. For kidney stones with a diameter greater than 2 cm, ESWL with double J stenting, PNL monotherapy, and lithotripsy using ureteroscopy are equally effective treatment choices, as well as for small-volume staghorn calculi.

Discussion

Because the JUA guidelines, especially those for staghorn calculi, were made using the same methodology as the AUA guidelines, the two guidelines resemble each other. It is difficult to perform prospective, randomized studies to compare several treatment modalities for staghorn calculi. After publication of the AUA clinical guidelines on staghorn calculi, Meretyk and his associates reported a prospective, randomized, single-center study involving 50 kidneys with complete staghorn calculi and compared ESWL monotherapy and combined treatment with PNL and ESWL. The stone-free rate was significantly greater and the complication rate was significantly lower in the combined PNL and ESWL treatment group. This is scientific evidence that combined PNL and ESWL should be recommended as the first-line treatment for most patients with staghorn calculi.

    The Health Care Office of the European Association of Urology (EAU) formulated common recommendations and guidelines for the treatment of patients with urolithiasis [21]. The recommended treatments for staghorn calculi, based on the EAU guidelines, depend on stone composition (Table 3). In selected cases of uric acid stones, combined treatment by ESWL and chemolysis might be useful. Although the EAU guidelines were clinically useful, we noted that the guidelines were produced mainly from the opinions of many experts rather than the results of meta-analysis.

TABLE 3. Active stone removal of complete and partial staghorn calculi[a]

Radio-opaque stones	1. PNL
	2. PNL → ESWL
	3. ESWL → PNL
	4. Open surgery
Infection stones	1. Antibiotics + PNL
	2. Antibiotics + PNL → ESWL
	3. Antibiotics + ESWL → PNL
	4. Antibiotics + open surgery
	5. Antibiotics + ESWL + chemolysis
Uric acid/urate stones	1. PNL
	2. PNL → ESWL
	2. PNL or ESWL + oral chemolysis
	3. ESWL → PNL
	4. Open surgery
Cystine stones	1. PNL
	2. PNL → ESWL
	3. ESWL → PNL
	4. Open surgery

[a] Tiselius et al. [21].

The treatment recommendations and results reported for the treatment of staghorn calculi are highly variable. One of the reasons for such varied results is the difficulty of accurately assessing the stone burden in patients with staghorn calculi. We need to research the clinical outcome of staghorn calculi using various treatment modalities with the same methods of describing the collecting system and the size of the staghorn calculi. The clinical efficacy and adverse events associated with the new extracorporeal shock wave lithotripters that are being used instead of the first-generation machines will need to be examined scientifically.

References

1. Libertino JA, Newman HR, Lytton B, Weiss RM (1971) Staghorn calculi in solitary kidneys. J Urol 105:753–757
2. Rous SN, Turner WR (1977) Retrospective study of 95 patients with staghorn calculus disease. J Urol 118:902–904
3. Koga S, Aratani Y, Matsuoka M, Ohyama C (1991) Staghorn calculi—long-term results of management. Br J Urol 68:122–124
4. Teichman JMH, Long RD, Hulbert JC (1995) Long-term renal fate and prognosis after staghorn calculus management. J Urol 153:1403–1407
5. Meno M, Parulkar BG, Drach GW (1998) Urinary lithiasis: etiology, diagnosis, and medical management. In: Walsh PC, et al. (eds) Campbell's urology, 7th edn. W. B. Saunders, Philadelphia, Vol. 3, Chapt. 91, pp 2661–2733
6. Segura JW, Preminger GM, Assimos DG, Dretler SP, Kahn RI, Lingeman JE, Macaluso JN, McCullough DL, Roehrborn CG, Bell H (1994) Nephrolithiasis Clini-

cal Guidelines Panel: report on the management of staghorn calculi. American Urological Association, Baltimore

7. Segura JW, Preminger GM, Assimos DG, Dretler SP, Kahn RI, Lingeman JE, Macaluso JN, McCullough DL (1994) Nephrolithiasis clinical guidelines panel summary report on the management of staghorn calculi. J Urol 151:1648–1651

8. Meretyk S, Goerit ON, Gafni O, Pode D, Shapiro A, Verstandig A, Sasson T, Katz G, Landau EH (1997) Complete staghorn calculi: random prospective comparison between extracorporeal shock wave lithotripsy monotherapy and combined with percutaneous nephrostolithotomy. J Urol 157:780–786

9. Winfield HN, Clayman RV, Chaussy CG, Weyman PJ, Fuchs GJ, Lupu AN (1988) Monotherapy of staghorn renal calculi: a comparative study between percutaneous nephrolithotomy and extracorporeal shock wave lithotripsy. J Urol 139:895–899

10. Lam HS, Lingeman JE, Barron M, Newman DM, Mosbaugh PG, Steele RE, Knapp PM, Scott JW, Nyhuis A, Woods JR (1992) Staghorn calculi: analysis of treatment results between initial percutaneous nephrostolithotomy and extracorporeal shock wave lithotripsy monotherapy with reference to surface area. J Urol 147:1219–1225

11. Lotti T, Caputo NA, Caggiano S, Zito A, Montanaro V, Papa S, Cancelmo G, Altieri V (1998) Possibilities and limits with the various treatment methods for large renal stones. Acta Urol Ital 12:137–141

12. Lingmann JE (1989) Relative roles of extracorporeal shock wave lithotripsy and percutaneous nephrolithotomy. In: Lingmann JE (ed) Shock wave lithotripsy, 2nd edn. Newmann, New York, pp 303–308

13. Bierkens AF, Hendrikx AJM, Lemmens WAJG, Debruyne FMJ (1991) Extracorporeal shock wave lithotripsy for large renal calculi: the role of ureteral stents. A randomized trial. J Urol 145:699–702

14. Netto NR, Lemos GC, Palma PCR, Fiuza L (1988) Staghorn calculi: percutaneous versus anatrophic nephrolithotomy. Eur Urol 15:9–12

15. Golijanin D, Katz R, Verstandig A, Sasson T, Laudau EH, Meretyk S (1998) The supracostal percutaneous nephrostomy for treatment of staghorn and complex kidney stones. J Endourol 12:403–405

16. Grasso M, Conlin M, Bagley D (1998) Retrograde ureteropyeloscopic treatment of 2 cm. or greater upper urinary tract and minor staghorn calculi. J Urol 160:346–351

17. Bruns T, Stein J, Tauber R (1995) Extracorporeal piezoelectric shock wave lithotripsy as mono and multiple therapy of large renal calculi including staghorn stones in unanaesthetized patients under semi-ambulant conditions. Br J Urol 75:435–440

18. Agrawal SP, Ridhorkar V, Naik D, Sabnis RB, Patel SH, Desai MR, Bapat SD (1998) Efficacy and safety of PCNL in solitary functioning kidneys with complex renal calculi. Indian J Urol 14:88–93

19. Rudnick DM, Bennett PM, Dretler SP (1999) Retrograde renoscopic fragmentation of moderate-size (1.5–3.0 cm) renal cystine stones. J Endourol 13:483–485

20. Morey AF, Nitahara KS, McAninch JW (1999) Modified anatrophic nephrolithotomy for management of staghorn calculi: Is renal function preserved? J Urol 162:670–673

21. Tiselius HG, Ackermann D, Alken P, Buck C, Conort P, Gallucci M (2001) Guidelines on urolithiasis. Eur Urol 40:362–371

Standard Treatment Modality for Ureteropelvic Junction Obstruction

Matthew T. Gettman and Joseph W. Segura

Summary. The standard treatment of ureteropelvic junction (UPJ) obstruction has radically changed. Whereas definitive management of UPJ obstruction previously required open surgery, endourologic and laparoscopic advances have increased the therapeutic possibilities. As new minimally invasive techniques have been introduced, the choice of therapy has become more complex and the preoperative evaluation has become more important. Indeed, the most appropriate treatment today must cater to characteristics of the individual patient. Open surgical procedures remain the gold standard of care; the other treatment options should strive for equivalent clinical success while improving quality of life and limiting disability. This chapter describes the clinical evaluation, treatment options, therapeutic concerns, and controversies regarding management of UPJ obstruction.

Key Words. Ureteropelvic junction obstruction, Pyeloplasty, Endopyelotomy, Acucise, Ureteroscopy, Laparoscopy

Introduction

With the introduction, success, and acceptance of minimally invasive techniques, management of ureteropelvic junction (UPJ) obstruction has radically changed. Although dismembered pyeloplasty remains the gold standard, minimally invasive procedures in properly selected patients can provide excellent success rates with decreased operative time and improved postoperative recovery [1]. In comparison to other endourologic treatments, antegrade endopyelotomy has consistently achieved success rates closest to those observed with open procedures [2–5]. Retrograde endopyelotomy, accompanied by advances in instrumentation, has increasingly become an accepted and successful treatment for

Department of Urology, Mayo Clinic, Mayo Building, East 17A, 200 First Street, S.W., Rochester, MN 55905, USA

UPJ obstruction [6–8]. In addition, laparoscopic management has yielded success rates similar to open surgery [9,10].

Indeed, the choice of intervention was easy when open surgery was the only option. Today, the most appropriate treatment must be selected on the basis of individual patient characteristics. Despite the appeal of endourologic and laparoscopic treatments, minimally invasive treatments should strive for success rates equivalent to those of open surgery while improving postoperative quality of life [1–10]. In this chapter we address the clinical evaluation, treatment options, therapeutic concerns, and controversies associated with UPJ obstruction.

Patient Evaluation

UPJ obstruction can present with a variety of complaints, including flank discomfort, urinary stones, hematuria, pyelonephritis, and renal dysfunction [11]. A thorough history and physical examination should be performed to uncover clues related to the diagnosis. Serum creatinine and routine urine studies are obtained for most patients. Classically, a patient will present with flank pain that is exacerbated by increased fluid intake and will have evidence of obstruction on excretory urogram. In this situation, additional workup prior to definitive treatment is infrequently required. For less straightforward cases, additional testing is required, which can include a diuretic renal scan, renal ultrasound, or, rarely today, a Whitaker pressure-perfusion test [1]. Retrograde pyelography is sometimes performed as the initial imaging test for patients with contrast allergies. In other instances, retrograde pyelography is completed as a confirmatory test prior to definitive treatment. We do not routinely assess patients with primary UPJ obstruction for the presence of crossing vessels.

While reviewing laboratory and imaging studies, identification of abnormalities such as marked hydronephrosis, poor renal function, renal anomalies, concurrent renal calculi, and high UPJ insertion is important, as these factors can influence treatment [2,6,12–21]. Endopyelotomy is contraindicated for patients with long avascular strictures (>2 cm), total obliteration of the UPJ, or severe periureteral fibrosis. A laparoscopic or open approach is warranted for these patients. A laparoscopic repair is contraindicated for most patients with a nondilated renal pelvis, recurrent pyelonephritis, or failed open pyeloplasty. Today, open surgical approaches are commonly reserved for patients not amenable to treatment with minimally invasive techniques. Other general contraindications to surgery include an uncorrected bleeding diathesis or untreated urinary tract infection. The risks and benefits of all treatments should be discussed with the patient. Ultimately, the choice of repair is dictated by anatomic characteristics, preference of the patient, and experience of the surgeon.

Treatment Options

Retrograde Endopyelotomy—Acucise

The Acucise cutting balloon catheter was approved in 1993 for treatment of UPJ obstruction. Retrograde endopyelotomy using the Acucise cutting balloon catheter represents the least invasive treatment for UPJ obstruction [6,7,15,2–30]. The Acucise method eliminates the need for percutaneous access to the UPJ and is the simplest of the available treatment options. The Acucise catheter can be placed across the UPJ obstruction using standard cystoscopic equipment, and a fine cutting wire precisely incises the obstruction. Since the Acucise procedure cannot be completed under direct visualization, the operative suite must have fluoroscopic equipment to monitor the surgical incision.

Complications are infrequently observed with the use of the Acucise device. In 12 series reported since 1993, the incidence of hemorrhagic complications was 4%, and the transfusion requirement was 3% [6,7,15,2–29]. Common sources of bleeding following Acucise endopyelotomy are injury to a lower-pole renal artery or renal parenchyma [22–29]. Other complications, including urinary tract infection, urinoma, and stent migration, have been reported [6,7,15,22–29].

In 11 series reported since 1993, the overall success rate was 77% (Table 1). Primary and secondary UPJ obstructions were effectively treated; the success rate for secondary obstruction (82%–100%) was slightly higher than that for primary obstruction (74%–81%) [6,7,15,22–29]. In a previous report by Brooks et al., the Acucise procedure was associated with a shorter recovery and less narcotic requirements than open pyeloplasty, laparoscopic pyeloplasty, or antegrade endopyelotomy [25]. In eight studies reporting hospitalization data, the mean length of stay ranged from 0.2 to 3 days [7,15,22,23,25,28,29]. Outpatient treatment is feasible with the Acucise technique. One concern is the high expense of the Acucise catheter, which is not reusable.

Retrograde Endopyelotomy—Ureteroscopic Technique

Inglis and Tolley described the first retrograde ureteroscopic endopyelotomy in 1986 [33]. With this method, the length, depth, and location of the surgical incision can be controlled under direct vision [8,13,34–40]. Similar to the Acucise procedure, the retrograde ureteroscopic approach eliminates risks associated with percutaneous access and the need for an external nephrostomy. The ureteroscopic method, however, requires much more technical skill than the Acucise method. Advances in ureteroscope design and instrumentation have simplified the ureteroscopic technique [35–38].

Complications reported with ureteroscopic endopyelotomy include hemorrhage, ureteral stricture, urinary tract infection, and stent migration [8,13,34–40]. In an early report by Meretyk et al., the incidence of ureteral strictures was 21% [34]. The high incidence of ureteral strictures was attributed to prolonged

TABLE 1. Results of Acucise endopyelotomy

Author	Year	Overall patients (UPJO)	Mean operative time (min)	Overall success rate (%)	Mean LOS (days)	Minor complication rate (%)	Major complication rate (%)	Mean follow-up (months)
Chandhoke [27]	1993	18	–	78 (14/18)	–	–	–	4
Anderson [28]	1995	25	62	84 (21/24)	1.7	16	0	8
Brooks [25]	1995	9	46	78 (7/9)	0.2	11	22	24
Cohen [24]	1996	9	42ᵃ	78 (7/9)	–	–	11	22
Nadler [7]	1996	26	63	81 (21/26)	1.6	4	0	33
Preminger [6]	1997	58 (66)	54	77 (43/56)	–	3	3	8
Gelet [26]	1997	44	53	76 (33/43)	6	–	14	12
Faerber [23]	1997	32 (36)	33	81 (26/32)	1.8	9	6	14
Gill [22]	1998	13	33	62 (8/13)	0.4	–	0	18
Kim [29]	1998	77	65	78 (60/77)	1.8	4	4 (3/77)	12
Lechevallier [15]	1999	36	30	75 (27/36)	3	22 (8/36)	8 (3/36)	24
Totals		351 (359)	48	77 (265/343)				15

UPJO, ureteropelvic junction obstruction; LOS, length of stay in hospital.
ᵃMean operative time based on 9 patients with UPJO and 6 patients with ureteral strictures.

operative times, the use of large-caliber ureteroscopes, and thermal injury from electrocautery. Thomas et al. advocated preoperative stent placement to permit passive ureteral dilation prior to ureteroscopic endopyelotomy [8,39]. Using this protocol, they achieved a success rate of 84% without stricture complications [39]. By using small-caliber ureteroscopes, retrograde endopyelotomy can now be completed without preoperative stenting. In five contemporary series using small-caliber ureteroscopes, none of the patients developed a stricture following treatment [14,35–38]. In eight reports published since 1990, only 1 of the 207 cumulative patients required a blood transfusion [8,13,34–38,40]. The reported incidence of minor complications (urinary tract infections, stent problem, etc.) in the same series ranged from 0% to 16% [8,13,34–38,40].

The overall success rate for eight series completed since 1990 was 84% (Table 2) [8,13,34–38,40]. The range of success rates was comparable for primary (82%–100%) and secondary (67%–100%) UPJ obstructions. However, surgical experience and follow-up are less with both retrograde techniques (ureteroscopic and Acucise) when compared with antegrade endopyelotomy (Tables 1–3). When compared with other minimally invasive treatments, ureteroscopic endopyelotomy (similar to Acucise) is associated with decreased narcotic and convalescence requirements [25,34]. In fact, many patients are treated as outpatients with this technique (Table 2).

Antegrade Endopyelotomy

Wickham and Kellet first described "percutaneous pyelolysis" in 1983 [41]. Smith modified and renamed the procedure as antegrade "endopyelotomy" in 1986 [42]. Antegrade endopyelotomy is an excellent choice when the UPJ is relatively dependent and no gross anatomic abnormalities are present [1,20,21]. In comparison to the other endourologic treatments, the surgical experience and success rates with antegrade endopyelotomy are the closest to those with open surgery [43–48]. Furthermore, follow-up for antegrade endopyelotomy is longer than that for other minimally invasive treatments [2,4,45]. Antegrade endopyelotomy does require expertise in percutaneous renal surgery [1]. After visualization of the UPJ, the endopyelotomy incision can be extended under direct vision with excellent precision. Excellent postoperative drainage is accomplished with a nephrostomy tube.

The complications of antegrade endopyelotomy are related to access or incision of the UPJ. Vascular injuries are the most worrisome [1]. In 14 larger series published since 1990, the incidence of severe bleeding requiring blood transfusion was 0%–8% [2–5,14,18,19,34,43–48]. In the same series, the incidence of urosepsis was 2%–4% (Table 3). Fluid absorption is less of a risk with endopyelotomy, since the operative time is typically less than the time required for percutaneous stone removal. Other rare complications associated with the procedure are ureteral necrosis, ureteral avulsion, pseudoaneurysm, arteriovenous fistula, urinoma, inadvertent incision of the renal pelvis, and stent migration [49–51].

TABLE 2. Results of retrograde ureteroscopic endopyelotomy

Author	Year	Patients	Size of ureteroscope	Modality for endopyelotomy	Mean operative time (min)	Success rate (%)	Mean LOS (days)	Minor complication rate (%)	Major complication rate (%)	Mean follow-up (months)
Clayman [40]	1990	10	9.8F, 10.8F, 12F	Cutting electrode	180	90 (9/10)	5	10		12
Meretyk [34]	1992	19	9.8F, 10.8F, 11F, 12F	Cutting electrode	179	79 (15/19)	3.4	16	37	17
Thomas [8]	1998	49	11.5F	Cutting electrode	90	84 (41/49)	1.2 (57% outpatient)	–	6 (3/49)	16
Tawfiek [35]	1998	32	6.9F, 7.5F, 9.8F	Cutting electrode, Ho:YAG laser	95	88 (28/32)	<1	3 (1/32)	0	62.5% ≥ 6 months 37.5% ≥ 12 months
Conlin [36]	1998	21	6.9F, 7.5F, 9.8F	Cutting electrode, Ho:YAG laser, cold knife	120[a]	81 (17/21)	–	15 (3/21)	0	23
Renner [13]	1998	34	8.5F	Nd:YAG	–	85 (29/34)	–	15 (5/34)	3 (1/34)	18
Gerber [38]	2000	22	6F, 8.5F	Cutting electrode, Ho:YAG laser	63	82 (18/22)	<24h in 21 patients	5 (1/22)	0	21[a]
Biyani [37]	2000	20 (22)	6.5F	Ho:YAG laser	44	85 (17/20)	1.9	5 (1/20)	5 (1/20)	34
Totals		207 (209)	–	–	107	84 (174/207)	–	–	–	20

[a] Median.

Table 3. Results of treatment with antegrade endopyelotomy

Author	Year	Patients (UPJO)	Modality for endopyelotomy	Mean operative time (min)	Success rate (%)	Mean LOS (days)	Transfusion rate (%)	Minor complication rate (%)	Major complication rate (%)	Mean follow-up (months)
Karlin [19]	1988	56	Cold hook knife	89	88 (49/56)	6.2	–	–	–	100% with 3+ months
Kuenkel [44]	1990	143	Cold knife	–	85 (121/143)	–	8 (11/143)	46	12 (17/143)	12
Cassis [43]	1991	27	Cold knife	–	78 (21/27)	–	0	33 (9/27)	11 (3/27)	3
Meretyk [34]	1992	23	Cold knife, cutting electrode	200	78 (18/23)	4	9 (2/23)	22	17	22
Perez [18]	1992	17	Cold knife	80	88 (15/17)	4	0 (0/17)	0	0	14
Motola [4]	1993	208 (212)	Cold hook knife	–	86 (182/212)	–	1 (2/208)	14 (29/208)	2 (5/208)	86% with 6+ months
Brooks [25]	1995	13	Cold hook knife	145	77 (10/13)	3	23 (3/13)	15	23	20
Kletscher [3]	1995	50	Cold straight knife	70[a]	88 (44/50)	3.8	4	0	6 (3/50)	12
Van Cangh [45]	1996	117	Cold knife	–	65 (56/86)	–	–	–	–	62
Gallucci [46]	1996	46	Cold straight and hook knife	–	80 (37/46)	–	2 (1/46)	52 (24/46)	4 (2/46)	100% with 12+ months
Korth [5]	1996	286	Cold knife	–	78 (183/236)	–	–	71 (168/236)	–	20
Combe [47]	1996	49	Cutting electrode	93	78 (38/49)	6.5	0	20 (10/49)	6 (3/49)	16
Gupta [2]	1997	393 (401)	Cold hook knife	–	85 (341/401)	–	–	–	–	51
Kahn [48]	1997	320	Cold hook knife	–	87 (278/320)	5	–	6 (20/320)	4 (14/320)	6+
Danuser [14]	1998	80	Cold hook knife	–	89 (71/80)	6	1.2 (1/80)	8 (6/80)	8 (6/80)	26
Totals		1828 (1840)	–	–	83 (1464/1759)	–	–	–	–	–

[a] Mean time also included percutaneous nephrostolithotomy in 14 cases.

99

Although antegrade endopyelotomy was initially used only for secondary obstruction [1–5], the procedure is currently effective for primary (success rates of 75%–90%) and secondary (success rates of 73%–91%) UPJ obstruction. In 15 series reported since 1988, the cumulative overall success rate was 83% (Table 3) [2–5,14,18,19,34,43–48].

In comparison to open surgery, antegrade endopyelotomy is less invasive, with decreased disability and earlier return to work [19]. The antegrade approach, however, is associated with a longer hospitalization and more discomfort than the other incisional techniques [25,34]. In an attempt to decrease discomfort from the nephrostomy tube and the length of hospitalization, a "tubeless" endopyelotomy and a mini-percutaneous endopyelotomy were recently described [52,53]. Bellman et al. reported a mean hospitalization time of 0.6 days for "tubeless" percutaneous renal surgery [52].

Laparoscopic Pyeloplasty

Laparoscopic pyeloplasty was introduced in 1993 to merge the high success rates of open pyeloplasty with the improved postoperative recovery of minimally invasive surgery [54]. Laparoscopic pyeloplasty is effective for patients with intrinsic obstruction, high insertion, a large renal pelvis, or crossing vessels [54–62]. From a technical standpoint, laparoscopic pyeloplasty is the most challenging treatment for UPJ obstruction. With the use of laparoscopic techniques, magnification enhances anatomic visualization of crossing vessels. In addition, the UPJ obstruction is managed by using plastic techniques developed for open pyeloplasty. Long operative times and increased surgical costs are the main disadvantages.

The rate of complications in 12 series reported since 1993 ranged from 5% to 27% (Table 4) [54–62]. Most complications were minor (transient flank pain, stent problems, superficial phlebitis, ileus); however, more significant complications (bowel injury, pulmonary embolus, urinoma) were reported. Hemorrhage was uncommon in the 12 series; 3 of 268 cumulative patients were noted to have a perinephric hematoma after surgery, but none required transfusion. In the same 12 series, open conversion was required in 5 of 268 cumulative patients (2%). The overall success rate was 97% for the 12 series published since 1993 (Table 4) [54–56]. As an alternative to a plastic repair for crossing vessels, Keeley et al. described laparoscopic division of crossing vessels in two patients [63]. The authors acknowledged that this approach was less than ideal and was indicated only when the crossing vessel supplied a small amount of parenchyma and no intrinsic narrowing was present [63].

Open Surgery

Open surgery remains the gold standard of treatment for UPJ obstruction. The advantages and disadvantages of open surgery have been previously described in detail [11,19,25,62,64,65]. Open surgery has been associated with success rates of 89% to 100% [11,19,25,62,64,65]. Currently, along with laparoscopic

Table 4. Results of laparoscopic pyeloplasty

Author	Year	Patients (UPJO)	Approach	Repair technique	Mean operative time (min)	Success rate (%)	Mean LOS (days)	Conversion rate (%)	Complication rate (%)	Mean follow-up (months)
Schuessler [54]	1993	5	Transperitoneal	Dismembered: 5	330	80 (4/5)	3	–	20	12
Recker [55]	1995	5	Transperitoneal	Dismembered: 5	305	100 (5/5)	8	20	–	–
Brooks [25]	1995	12	Transperitoneal	Dismembered: 12	356	100 (12/12)	3.1	–	25	14
Nakada [56]	1995	4	Transperitoneal	Dismembered: 3 Culp-DeWeerd: 1	530	100 (4/4)	4	–	–	–
Janetschek [9]	1996	17	Combined: 14 Retroperitoneal: 3	Dismembered: 8 Ureterolysis: 4 Y-V plasty: 3 End-to-end: 1	280	100 (17/17)	7	11	11	–
Chen [57]	1996	13	Transperitoneal	Dismembered: 13	340	100 (13/13)	3.2	–	15	13
Moore [58]	1997	29 (30)	Transperitoneal	Dismembered: 26 Y-V plasty: 4	270	97 (29/30)	3.4	–	14	–
Chen [59]	1998	57	Transperitoneal	Dismembered: 44 Y-V plasty: 13	258	94 (32/34)	3.3	0	12 (7/57)	17
Bauer [10]	1999	42	Transperitoneal	Dismembered, Y-V plasty	–	98 (41/42)	–	0	12	15
Ben Slama [60]	2000	15	Retroperitoneal	Dismembered: 8 Fenger plasty: 7	178	93 (14/15)	4.8	7	28 (4/15)	17
Janetschek [61]	2000	65 (67)	Transperitoneal: 59 Retroperitoneal: 7	Fenger plasty: 63 Y-V plasty: 4	119	98 (64/65)	4.1	2	3 (2/65)	25
Soulie [62]	2001	25 (26)	Retroperitoneal	Dismembered: 24 Y-V plasty: 2	165	92 (24/26)	4.5	4	11.5	3
Totals	–	289 (293)	–	–	285	97 (259/268)	–	–	–	15

pyeloplasty, open surgery provides the highest success rates for treatment of UPJ obstruction. Use of open UPJ repair has substantially decreased with the introduction of endourologic and laparoscopic procedures. In fact, open UPJ repair is commonly reserved for patients for whom minimally invasive treatments have failed or who have contraindications to such techniques.

Therapeutic Concerns

Renal Function

Poor renal function can adversely impact management of UPJ obstruction with endopyelotomy. Gupta et al. reviewed the patient records from 60 failed antegrade endopyelotomies over a 12-year period [2]. Split renal function was determined by renal scans and stratified into poor (<25%), moderate (25%–40%), and good (>40%) function. The success rate for patients with poor renal function was significantly worse (success rate of 54%) than for those with moderate (80% success) or good (92% success) renal function. For patients undergoing ureteroscopic endopyelotomy, Biyani et al. also reported the adverse effect of poor renal function (split renal function <25%). In the report, all patients with renal function <25% had an unsatisfactory result at a mean follow-up of 34 months [37].

When renal function from the obstructed kidney is <25% and the opposite kidney is normal, the patient should be informed that treatment with endopyelotomy is less successful. Rather than take the risk of endoscopic failure, some patients may choose a dismembered procedure (laparoscopic or open) or even a laparoscopic nephrectomy. If the involved kidney has substantial renal parenchyma, a trial of percutaneous drainage with repeat renal scan is indicated before proceeding with nephrectomy.

Hydronephrosis

High-grade hydronephrosis has adversely impacted definitive management of UPJ obstruction in prior reports [2,13,14,66]. In 102 patients treated with antegrade endopyelotomy, Van Cangh et al. reported a 95% success rate for patients with grade 1 or 2 hydronephrosis and no crossing vessels, whereas similar patients with grade 3 or 4 hydronephrosis had success rates of 77% [66]. For patients treated with retrograde ureteroscopic endopyelotomy, Renner et al. reported that high-grade hydonephrosis was the only factor that predicted treatment failure [13]. Gupta et al. also reported that high-grade hydronephrosis adversely impacted treatment with antegrade endopyelotomy. Patients with massive hydronephrosis had a 50% success rate, compared with a 96% success rate for those with moderate hydronephrosis [2]. Danuser et al. measured pyelocaliceal volume in 75 of 80 patients undergoing antegrade endopyelotomy [14]. The probability of successful endopyelotomy was better for patients with a volume <50ml (87% success rate) and worse for patients with a volume >50ml (76%

success rate) [14]. For Acucise endopyelotomy, Lechavallier et al. reported that hydronephrosis did not impact treatment [15]. Instead, they noted that only crossing vessels portended an adverse outcome on multivariate analysis.

For patients undergoing dismembered pyeloplasty (open or laparoscopic), the degree of hydronephrosis alone is not a significant cause for concern, since the UPJ can be remodeled during repair. Conversely, endopyelotomy can effectively relieve intrinsic obstruction, but remodeling of the UPJ is impossible.

Concurrent Stone Disease

Antegrade endopyelotomy is favored for patients with UPJ obstruction and concurrent renal stones; however, open and laparoscopic approaches are equally effective in selected patients [1–5]. In addition, stone removal is possible with retrograde ureteroscopic endopyelotomy; however, Acucise endopyelotomy is contraindicated for patients with concurrent stones.

For mobile stones without mucosal edema, percutaneous stone removal followed by immediate endopyelotomy provides excellent treatment [1,3]. If the stone burden has created significant mucosal edema that casts doubt on the validity of the UPJ obstruction, antegrade stone removal followed by radiographic re-evaluation of the UPJ is sometimes indicated before proceeding with endopyelotomy.

The etiology of renal stones associated with UPJ obstruction is debatable. Husmann et al. noted that 76% of patients with nonstruvite stones had identifiable metabolic abnormalities [67]. Futhermore, the rate of stone recurrence was significantly reduced if patients underwent pyeloplasty and medical stone treatment versus pyeloplasty alone. Matin and Streem recently confirmed that metabolic abnormalities predispose patients to stone formation with UPJ obstruction [68]. On the other hand, Bernardo et al. found a low incidence of recurrence and metabolic abnormalities following endopyelotomy [69]. They suggested that correction of the anatomic obstruction alone decreased the risk of stone recurrence.

Patient Age

Age is not an absolute contraindication to endoscopic or laparoscopic management of UPJ obstruction, except in small children. All patients must be suitable candidates for either regional or general anesthesia. Patient size also does not preclude the use of endoscopic or laparoscopic procedures. For children under 6 years of age, open surgery remains the first-line treatment of UPJ obstruction and yields success rates over 90% [61,65,70].

Little information has been reported on the use of minimally invasive treatments in the pediatric population. In 22 patients from two studies, antegrade endopyelotomy for primary obstruction achieved a 68% success rate [72,73]. In 17 patients from four studies, the success rate for treatment of secondary UPJ obstruction was 94% [72–75]. Acucise endopyelotomy was reported in 8 children (age 4–15 years) and achieved an 88% success rate with a mean follow-up of 15 months [76]. Although laparoscopic pyeloplasty has been reported in a 3-month-old infant, the youngest patients treated by Janetschek et al. and Bauer et al. were 11 and 12 years old, respectively [10,61]. The role of minimally invasive treatments in the pediatric population remains to be defined.

Renal Anomalies

The presence of UPJ obstruction in anomalous kidneys can increase the complexity of treatment. UPJ obstruction is associated with 15%–33% of horseshoe kidneys and up to 22% of ectopic kidneys [77,78]. Historically, the success rates for open repair of anomalous kidneys are 55%–80% [79,80]. Information regarding endourologic or laparoscopic treatment of UPJ obstruction in anomalous kidneys is limited. Jabbour et al. evaluated the use of antegrade endopyelotomy for horseshoe (four patients), lumbar ectopic (three patients), and pelvic (two patients) kidneys [16]. An overall success rate of 78% was noted, with a mean follow-up of 62 months [16]. Percutaneous access for the pelvic kidneys was obtained with laparoscopic assistance. Other investigators have also treated horseshoe kidneys with antegrade endopyelotomy [17,81]. Janetschek et al. treated one horseshoe kidney with laparoscopic pyeloplasty [61], and Conlin et al. successfully used ureteroscopic endopyelotomy [36]. Jabbour et al. recommended that the Acucise method not be used for treatment of UPJ obstruction in anomalous kidneys [16]. Also, preoperative assessment of crossing vessels does appear warranted before endourologic management of UPJ obstruction in anomalous kidneys is undertaken.

High-Insertion UPJ Obstruction

Historically, high-insertion UPJ obstruction was thought to adversely impact treatment with endourologic techniques and require management with dismembered pyeloplasty or Y-V plasty. In prior reports, investigators preferred endopyelotomy when the UPJ obstruction was dependent [1,18,21]. Perez et al. suggested that high-insertion UPJ obstruction compromised endourologic treatment and contributed to treatment failure with antegrade endopyelotomy [18].

On the other hand, Karlin et al. suggested that antegrade endopyelotomy was feasible for patients with high insertion [19]. In addition, Shalhav et al. used Acucise or antegrade endopyelotomy to treat 10 patients with high insertion [21]. The subjective success rate for the 10 patients was 80%, with a mean follow-up of 27 months, whereas the objective success rate was 70%, with a mean follow-up of 26 months. Moreover, Shalhav et al. combined data from recent series and noted a 78% success rate for 19 patients with high-insertion UPJ obstruction [21]. In the combined group, antegrade endopyelotomy was 90% successful (9 of 10 patients), whereas Acucise was 68% successful (5 of 8 patients). Likewise, Chow et al. studied 19 patients with high insertion treated with antegrade or Acucise endopyelotomy and reported an overall 79% success rate [20]. Based on available reports, endopyelotomy does appear effective for patients with high insertion; however, endopyelotomy is still associated with better success rates when the UPJ is dependent [1].

Treatment Controversies

Evaluation of Crossing Vessels

The preoperative evaluation of crossing vessels for patients with primary UPJ obstruction is controversial. For patients undergoing open or laparoscopic management, a workup is not warranted. For patients treated with endopyelotomy (antegrade, retrograde urteroscopic, retrograde Acucise), the workup is highly debated. At a mean follow-up of 5 years, Van Cangh et al. prospectively studied the success rates for 67 patients evaluated with preoperative angiograms and treated with antegrade endopyelotomy [66]. Patients with a combination of crossing vessels on angiogram and high-grade hydronephrosis had a 39% success rate, versus a 95% success rate for patients without either abnormality [66]. In a similar investigation, Van Cangh et al. reported that crossing vessels were more common with endopyelotomy failures (67%) than with successful cases (18%) [45]. On the other hand, Gupta et al. reported an 85% success rate for 401 antegrade endopyelotomies. Of the 60 treatment failures, 54 patients underwent open exploration and repair. The most common findings were extrinsic fibrosis and intrinsic stenosis. Crossing vessels were identified in only 13 patients, suggesting that this factor contributed to treatment failure in only 4% of cases [2]. In addition, Nakada et al. completed spiral CT angiograms on 16 patients successfully treated with Acucise endopyelotomy with more than 2 years follow-up [82]. Among the 16 patients, 38% had anterior or posterior crossing vessels, despite successful outcomes [82].

Some investigators have suggested that an evaluation of crossing vessels is warranted not only to improve endopyelotomy outcome, but also to avoid a potential source of perioperative complications. However, Sampaio and Favorito have extensively studied the vascular anatomy surrounding the kidney, noting that 71% of patients have a vessel within 1.5 cm of the UPJ [83]. More importantly, the majority or blood vessels are located anterior (91%) or posterior (approximately 9%), but rarely lateral to the UPJ [83]. Based on this knowledge alone, a lateral endopyelotomy can be confidently completed in most instances without the need for an expensive radiologic evaluation of crossing vessels. For instance, after modifying the location of the incision from a posterolateral to a due lateral position, Kim et al. observed no hemorrhagic complications with Acucise endopyelotomy [29].

Obviously, the location of the endopyelotomy is more problematic for patients with an ectopic kidney, malrotated kidney, or secondary UPJ obstruction. Advanced imaging techniques (spiral CT and endoluminal ultrasound) have simplified the preoperative evaluation of crossing vessels, and therefore an evaluation of crossing vessels is prudent for high-risk patients.

Stenting

The optimal duration of stenting and stent size following endopyelotomy is controversial. Based on the work of Davis, the stent is a crucial element for healing after ureteral incision. In the canine model, Davis reported a 90% regeneration of ureteral musculature 6 weeks after intubated ureterotomy [84]. Later, Oppenheimer and Hinman reported that 8–12 weeks was required for full regeneration of ureteral musculature, and 1 week was required for urothelial regeneration [85]. Based on these data, a 6-week duration of stenting has become the gold standard following endopyelotomy.

Experimental and clinical evidence suggests that stents may not be required for the entire duration of healing following endopyelotomy. Kerbl et al. noted that healing after Acucise endoureterotomy was equivalent after 1, 3, or 6 weeks of stenting [86]. In fact, healing was better at 1 week for strictures >2 cm in length. Clinically, Kuenkel and Korth retrospectively compared a stent duration of 3 weeks (113 patients) to 6 weeks (30 patients) following antegrade endopyelotomy [44]. At a mean follow-up of 12.4 months, the success rate was 78% in the 3-week group and 60% in the 6-week group [44]. Kumar et al. additionally noted equivalent success rates at 1 year of follow-up for patients receiving stents for 2 weeks (13 patients) or 4 weeks (13 patients) after antegrade endopyelotomy [87]. Although earlier stent removal may be feasible, a prospective evaluation appears warranted to further evaluate optimal stent duration.

Based on the routine use of 12–16 F splints for intubated ureterotomy [84], large-caliber graduated endopyelotomy stents were initially favored after endopyelotomy. These stents were very difficult to place in the previously unstented ureter and did not appear to improve the success rate [1–3]. For instance, Kletscher et al. achieved a 95% success for 21 patients receiving an 8 F or 8.5 F stent, compared with a 85% success for 26 patients receiving a 14 F/7 F endopyelotomy stent following an antegrade endopyelotomy [3]. Currently, the trend is to use smaller-caliber stents that are less expensive and easier to place. Prospective, randomized trials would also help resolve issues of stent size after endopyelotomy.

Comparisons of Treatment

Previous reports have compared treatment modalities for UPJ obstruction. Shalhav et al. retrospectively compared the results of antegrade endopyelotomy (83 patients) and Acucise endopyelotomy (66 patients) [88]. Overall, the Acucise procedure required a significantly shorter operative time and hospitalization. In patients with primary UPJ obstruction, the success rate was 89% for antegrade endopyelotomy and 71% for the Acucise technique. For secondary UPJ obstructions, the success rate was 77% for antegrade endopyelotomy and 83% for Acucise. However, in primary and secondary endopyelotomy, the Acucise method was 20% and 37% more cost effective, respectively [88].

Meretyk et al. compared antegrade endopyelotomy (23 patients) with retrograde ureteroscopic endopyelotomy (19 patients) in a retrospective report using large-caliber ureteroscopes without prestenting [34]. At a mean follow-up of 9.5 months for antegrade and 12 months for retrograde endopyelotomy, the objective success rates were 78% and 79%, respectively. However, prolonged operative time and large-caliber scopes were thought to contribute to the 21% delayed stricture rate in the group undergoing retrograde endopyelotomy [34]. To date, comparative studies with smaller-caliber ureteroscopes have not been completed.

Karlin et al. retrospectively compared antegrade endopyelotomy (56 patients) with open pyeloplasty (32 patients) early in the era of endourologic management of UPJ obstruction [19]. The endopyelotomy required less operative time, fewer narcotics, fewer hospital days, and shorter convalescence after surgery. Endopyelotomy was 87.5% successful, whereas open pyeloplasty was 95%–98% successful [19].

Soulie et al. prospectively compared laparoscopic pyeloplasty with open pyeloplasty for 53 nonrandomized patients treated between 1997 and 2000 [62]. The mean length of the surgical incision in the group undergoing open pyeloplasty was 5 cm. At 3-month follow-up, the success rates for laparoscopic and open pyeloplasty were 88.5% and 89.3%, respectively. Hospitalization, operative time, blood loss, and complication rates were equivalent between groups; however, return to painless activity was faster with laparoscopic treatment [62].

Brooks et al. retrospectively compared open pyeloplasty with antegrade endopyelotomy, Acucise endopyelotomy, and laparoscopic pyeloplasty for 45 patients treated between 1990 and 1994 [25]. The success rates were 100% for open and laparoscopic pyeloplasty, 78% for Acucise endopyelotomy, and 77% for antegrade endopyelotomy. Complications were similar among all groups. The convalescence was shorter for Acucise endopyelotomy (1 week) than for laparoscopic pyeloplasty (2.3 weeks), antegrade endopyelotomy (4.7 weeks), or open pyeloplasty (10.3 weeks) [25].

Conclusions

With the introduction of minimally invasive treatments, definitive management of UPJ obstruction must be tailored to the preference of the individual patient, the anatomic characteristics of the patient, and the surgical expertise of the urologist. Although open surgery remains the gold standard of treatment, minimally invasive procedures are warranted as first-line treatments for most patients.

At our institution, the favored approach is antegrade endopyelotomy. The retrograde ureteroscopic approach is a good alternative; however, even with advanced instrumentation this technique can be cumbersome. The Acucise technique is less appealing because of the blind nature of the incision. In the current era, the laparoscopic approach has definite advantages in comparison with open surgery.

Standardization of treatment for UPJ obstruction is difficult, because many factors influence the outcome. Prospective, randomized studies may help delineate a standard treatment modality for UPJ obstruction; however, the validity of such studies may be doubtful, given the complexity of issues guiding therapeutic recommendations.

References

1. Segura JW (1998) Antegrade endopyelotomy. Urol Clin N Am 25:311–316
2. Gupta M, Tuncay OT, Smith AD (1997) Open surgical exploration after failed endopyelotomy: a 12-year perspective. J Urol 157:1613–1619
3. Kletscher BA, Segura JW, LeRoy AJ, Patterson DE (1995) Percutaneous antegrade endopyelotomy: review of 50 consecutive cases. J Urol 153:701–703
4. Motola JA, Badlani GH, Smith AD (1993) Results of 212 consecutive endopyelotomies: an 8-year followup. J Urol 149:453–456
5. Korth K, Kuenkel M, Karsch J (1996) Percutaneous endopyelotomy and results: Korth technique. J Endourol 10:121–126
6. Preminger GM, Clayman RV, Nakada SY, Babayan RK, Albala DM, Fuchs GJ, Smith AD (1997) A multicenter clinical trial investigating the use of a fluoroscopically controlled cutting balloon catheter for the management of ureteral and ureteropelvic junction obstruction. J Urol 157:1625–1629
7. Nadler RB, Rao GS, Pearle MS, Nakada SY, Clayman RV (1996) Acucise endopyelotomy: assessment of long-term durability. J Urol 156:1094–1097
8. Thomas R, Monga M (1998) Endopyelotomy retrograde ureteroscopic approach. Urol Clin N Am 25:305–310
9. Janetschek G, Peschel R, Altarac S, Bartsch G (1996) Laparoscopic and retroperitoneoscopic repair of ureteropelvic junction obstruction. Urology 47:311–316
10. Bauer JJ, Bishoff JT, Moore RG, Chen RN, Iverson AJ, Kavoussi LR (1999) J Urol 162:692–695
11. Clark WR, Malek RS (1987) Ureteropelvic junction obstruction. I. Observations on the classic type in adults. J Urol 138:276–279
12. Van Cangh PJ, Wilmart JF, Opsomer RJ, Abi-Aad A, Wese FX, Lorge F (1994) Long-term results and late recurrence after endoureteropyelotomy: a critical analysis of prognostic factors. J Urol 151:934–937
13. Renner C, Frede T, Seemann O, Rassweiler J (1998) Laser endopyelotomy: minimally invasive therapy of ureteropelvic junction stenosis. J Endourol 12:537–544
14. Danuser H, Ackermann DK, Bohlen D, Studer UE (1998) Endopyelotomy for primary ureteropelvic junction obstruction: risk factors determine the success rate. J Urol 159:56–61
15. Lechevallier E, Eghazarian C, Ortega J, Andre M, Gelsi E, Coulange C (1999) Retrograde Acucise endopyelotomy: long-term results. J Endourol 13:575–580
16. Jabbour ME, Goldfischer ER, Stravodimos KG, Klima WJ, Smith AD (1998) Endopyelotomy for horseshoe and ectopic kidneys. J Urol 160:694–697
17. Bellman GC, Yamaguchi R (1996) Special considerations in endopyelotomy in a horseshoe kidney. Urology 47:582–586
18. Perez LM, Friedman RM, Carson CC III (1992) Endopyelotomy in adults. Urology 39:71–76

19. Karlin GS, Badlani GH, Smith AD (1988) Endopyelotomy versus open pyeloplasty: comparison in 88 patients. J Urol 140:476–478
20. Chow GK, Geisinger MA, Streem SB (1999) Endopyelotomy outcome as a function of high versus dependent ureteral insertion. Urology 54:999–1002
21. Shalhav AL, Giusti G, Elbahnasy AM, Hoenig DM, Maxwell KL, McDougall EM, Clayman RV (1998) Endopyelotomy for high insertion ureteropelvic junction obstruction. J Endourol 12:127–130
22. Gill HS, Liao JC (1998) Pelvi-ureteric junction obstruction treated with acucise retrograde endopyelotomy. Br J Urol 82:8–11
23. Faerber GJ, Richardson TD, Farah N, Ohl DA (1997) Retrograde treatment of ureteropelvic junction obstruction using the ureteral cutting balloon catheter. J Urol 157:454–458
24. Cohen TD, Gross MB, Preminger GM (1996) Long-term follow-up of Acucise incision of ureteropelvic junction obstruction and ureteral strictures. Urology 47:317–323
25. Brooks JD, Kavoussi LR, Preminger GM, Schuessler WW, Moore RG (1995) Comparison of open and endourologic approaches to the obstructed ureteropelvic junction. Urology 46:791–795
26. Gelet A, Combe M, Ramackers JM, Ben Rais N, Martin X, Dawahra M, Marechal JM, Dubernard JM (1997) Endopyelotomy with the Acucise cutting balloon device. Eur Urol 31:389–393
27. Chandhoke PS, Clayman RV, Stone AM, McDougall EM, Buelna T, Hilal N, Chang M, Stegwell MJ (1993) Endopyelotomy and endoureterotomy with the Acucise ureteral cutting balloon device: preliminary experience. J Endourol 7:45–51
28. Anderson KR, Clayman RV (1995) Acucise endopyelotomy. In: Smith AD (ed) Controversies in endourology. W.B. Saunders, London, p 274
29. Kim FJ, Herrell SD, Jahoda AE, Albala DM (1998) Complications of Acucise endopyelotomy. J Endourol 12:433–436
30. Schwartz BF, Stoller ML (1999) Complications of retrograde balloon cautery endopyelotomy. J Urol 162:1594–1598
31. Wagner JR, D'Agostino R, Babayan RK (1996) Renal arterioureteral hemorrhage: a complication of Acucise endopyelotomy. Urology 48:139–141
32. Streem SB, Geisinger MA (1995) Prevention and management of hemorrhage associated with cautery wire balloon incision of ureteropelvic junction obstruction. J Urol 153:1904–1906
33. Inglis JA, Tolley DA (1986) Ureteroscopic pyelosis for pelviureteric junction obstruction. Br J Urol 58:250–252
34. Meretyk I, Meretyk S, Clayman RV (1992) Endopyelotomy: comparison of ureteroscopic retrograde and antegrade percutaneous techniques. J Urol 148:775–783
35. Tawfiek ER, Liu J, Bagley DH (1998) Ureteroscopic treatment of ureteropelvic junction obstruction. J Urol 160:1643–1647
36. Conlin MJ, Bagley DH (1998) Ureteroscopic endopyelotomy at a single setting. J Urol 159:77–731
37. Biyani CS, Cornford PA, Powell CS (2000) Ureteroscopic endopyelotomy with the holmium:YAG laser. Eur Urol 38:139–143
38. Gerber GS, Kim JC (2000) Ureteroscopic endopyelotomy in the treatment of patients with ureteropelvic junction obstruction. Urology 55:198–202
39. Thomas R, Monga M, Klein EW (1996) Ureteroscopic retrograde endopyelotomy for management of ureteropelvic junction obstruction. J Endourol 10:141–145

40. Clayman RV, Basler JW, Kavoussi L, Picus DD (1990) Ureteroscopic endopyelotomy. J Urol 144:246–252

41. Wickham JEA, Kellet MJ (1983) Percutaneous pyelosis. Eur Urol 9:122–124

42. Badlani G, Eshghi M, Smith AD (1986) Percutaneous surgery for ureteropelvic junction obstruction (endopyelotomy): technique and early results. J Urol 135:26–28

43. Cassis AN, Brannen GE, Bush WH, Correa RJ, Chambers M (1991) Endopyelotomy: review of results and complications. J Urol 146:1492–1495

44. Kuenkel M, Korth K (1990) Endopyelotomy: long-term follow-up of 143 patients. J Endourol 4:109–116

45. Van Cangh PJ, Nesa S, Galeon M, Tombal B, Wese FX, Dardenne AN, Opsomer R, Lorge F (1996) Vessels around the ureteropelvic junction: significance and imaging by conventional radiology. J Endourol 10:111–119

46. Gallucci M, Alpi G (1996) Antegrade transpelvic endopyelotomy in primary obstruction of the ureteropelvic junction. J Endourol 10:127–132

47. Combe M, Gelet A, Abdelrahim AF, Lopez JG, Dawahra M, Martin X, Marechal JM, Dubernard JM (1996) Ureteropelvic invagination procedure for endopyelotomy (Gelet technique): review of 51 consecutive cases. J Endourol 10:153–157

48. Khan AM, Holman E, Pasztor I, Toth C (1997) Endopyelotomy: experience with 320 cases. J Endourol 11:243–246

49. Bellman GC (1996) Complications of endopyelotomy. J Endourol 10:177–181

50. Sutherland RS, Pfister RR, Koyle MA (1992) Endopyelotomy associated ureteral necrosis: complete ureteral replacement using the Boari flap. J Urol 148:1490–1492

51. Malden ES, Picus D, Clayman RV (1992) Arteriovenous fistula complicating endopyelotomy. J Urol 148:1520–1523

52. Bellman GC, Davidoff R, Candela J, Gerspach J, Kurtz S, Stout L (1997) Tubeless percutaneous renal surgery. J Urol 157:1578–1582

53. Monga M (1999) Mini-percutaneous antegrade endopyelotomy. Tech Urol 5:223–225

54. Schuessler WW, Grune MT, Tecuanhuey LV, Preminger GM (1993) Laparoscopic dismembered pyeloplasty. J Urol 150:1795–1799

55. Recker F, Subotic B, Geopel M, Tscholl R (1995) Laparoscopic dismembered pyeloplasty: preliminary report. J Urol 153:1601–1604

56. Nakada SY, McDougall EM, Clayman RV (1995) Laparoscopic pyeloplasty for secondary ureteropelvic junction obstruction: preliminary experience. Urology 46:257–260

57. Chen RN, Moore RG, Kavoussi LR (1996) Laparoscopic pyeloplasty. J Endourol 10:159–161

58. Moore RG, Averch TD, Schulam PG, Adams JB, Chen RN, Kavoussi LR (1997) Laparoscopic pyeloplasty: experience with the initial 30 cases. J Urol 157:459–462

59. Chen RN, Moore RG, Kavoussi LR (1998) Laparoscopic pyeloplasty indications, technique, and long-term outcome. Urol Clin N Am 25:323–330

60. Ben Slama MR, Salomon L, Hoznek A, Cicco A, Saint F, Alame W, Antiphon P, Chopin DK, Abbou CC (2000) Extraperitoneal laparoscopic repair of ureteropelvic junction obstruction: initial experience in 15 cases. Urology 56:45–48

61. Janetschek G, Reschel R, Franscher F (2000) Laparoscopic pyeloplasty. Urol Clin N Am 27:695–704

62. Soulie M, Thoulouzan M, Seguin P, Mouly P, Vazzoler N, Pontonnier F, Plante P (2001) Retroperitoneal laparoscopic versus open pyeloplasty with a minimal incision: comparison of two surgical approaches. Urology 57:443–447

63. Keeley FX, Bagley DH, Kulp-Hugues D, Gomella LG (1996) Laparoscopic division of crossing vessels at the ureteropelvic junction. J Endourol 10:163–168
64. Streem SB (1998) Ureteropelvic junction obstruction open operative intervention. Urol Clin N Am 25:331–341
65. Lim DJ, Walker RD III (1996) Management of the failed pyeloplasty. J Urol 156: 738–740
66. Van Cangh PJ, Wilmart JF, Opsomer RJ, Abi-Aad A, Wese FX, Lorge F (1994) Long-term results and late recurrence after endoureteropyelotomy: a critical analysis of prognostic factors. J Urol 151:934–937
67. Husmann DA, Milliner DS, Segura JW (1995) Ureteropelvic junction obstruction with a simultaneous renal calculus: long-term follow up. J Urol 153:1399–1402
68. Matin SF, Streem SB (2000) Metabolic risk factors in patients with ureteropelvic junction obstruction and renal calculi. J Urol 163:1676–1678
69. Bernardo NO, Liatsikos EN, Dinlenc CZ, Kapoor R, Fogarty JD, Smith AD (2000) Stone recurrence after endopyelotomy. Urology 56:378–381
70. Goldfischer ER, Smith AD (1998) Endopyelotomy revisited. Urology 51:855–857
71. Lim DJ, Walker RD III (1996) Management of failed pyeloplasty. J Urol 156:738–740
72. Figenshau RS, Clayman RV, Colberg JW, Coplen DE, Soble JJ, Manley CB (1996) Pediatric endopyelotomy: the Washington University experience. J Urol 156: 2025–2030
73. Tan HL, Najmaldin A, Webb DR (1993) Endopyelotomy for pelvi-ureteric junction obstruction in children. Eur Urol 24:84–88
74. Kavoussi LR, Meretyk S, Dierks SM, Biggs SW, Gup DI, Manley CB, Shapiro E, Clayman RV (1991) Endopyelotomy for secondary ureteropelvic junction obstruction in children. J Urol 145:345–349
75. Faerber GJ, Ritchey ML, Bloom DA (1995) Percutaneous endopyelotomy in infants and young children after failed open pyeloplasty. J Urol 154:1495–1497
76. Bogaert GA, Kogan BA, Mevorach RA, Stoller ML (1996) Efficacy of retrograde endopyelotomy in children. J Urol 156:734–737
77. Segura JW, Kelalis PP, Burke EC (1972) Horseshoe kidney in children. J Urol 108: 333–336
78. Gleason PE, Kelalis PP, Husmann DA, Kramer SA (1994) Hydronephrosis in renal ectopia: incidence, etiology, and significance. J Urol 151:1660–1661
79. Culp OS, Winterringer JR (1955) Surgical treatment of horseshoe kidney: comparison of results after various types of operations. J Urol 73:747–756
80. Pitts WR Jr, Muecke EC (1975) Horseshoe kidneys: a 40-year experience. J Urol 113: 743–746
81. Nakamura K, Baba S, Tazaki H (1994) Endopyelotomy in horseshoe kidneys. J Endourol 8:203–206
82. Nakada SY, Wolf JS Jr, Brink JA, Quillen SP, Nadler RB, Gaines MV, Clayman RV (1998) Retrospective analysis of the effect of crossing vessels on successful retrograde endopyelotomy outcomes using spiral computerized tomography angiography. J Urol 159:62–65
83. Sampaio FJB, Favorito LA (1993) Ureteropelvic junction stenosis: vascular anatomical background for endopyelotomy. J Urol 150:1787–1791
84. Davis DM, Strong GH, Drake WM (1943) Intubated ureterotomy: a new operation for ureteral and ureteral pelvic strictures. Surg Gynecol Obset 76:513–523
85. Oppenheimer R, Hinman F Jr (1955) Ureteral regeneration: contracture vs. hyperplasia of smooth muscle. J Urol 74:476–484

86. Kerbl K, Chandhoke PS, Figenshau RS, Stone AM, Clayman RV (1993) Effect of stent duration on ureteral healing following endoureterotomy in an animal model. J Urol 150:1302–1305

87. Kumar R, Kapoor R, Mandhani A, Kumar A, Ahlawat R (1999) Optimum duration of splinting after endopyelotomy. J Endourol 13:89–92

88. Shalhav AL, Giusti G, Elbahnasy AM, Hoenig DM, McDougall EM, Smith DS, Maxwell KL, Clayman RV (1998) Adult endopyelotomy: impact of etiology and antegrade versus retrograde approach on outcome. J Urol 160:685–689

Standard Treatment Modality for Female Stress Incontinence

Osamu Nishizawa[1], Yoko Yoshikawa[2], Momokazu Gotoh[2], and Maki Nakata[3]

Summary. The treatment modalities for female stress incontinence include physiotherapy, drug therapy, surgical treatment, and the use of absorbents, and devices. In general, physiotherapy is selected first for mild to moderate cases. The efficacy of drug therapy for stress incontinence has not been evaluated in a randomized, controlled trial, such that drug therapy is currently positioned as a supplemental treatment. Surgical treatment is used in moderate to severe cases. Surgical treatment can be classified into five categories: retropubic suspension, transvaginal suspension, sling operation, anterior repair, and periurethral injection of bulking agents. Meta-analytical results of a long-term study (4 years or more) showed that the rates of elimination of incontinence were 84% for retropubic suspension, 67% for transvaginal suspension, 83% for sling operation, and 61% for anterior repair. Retropubic suspension and sling operation were more effective than the other surgical techniques. Major complications in surgical treatment include urinary disturbance due to urethral obstruction and postoperative de novo urgency. Meta-analysis showed that the frequency of urinary retention was about 5% after transvaginal suspension and about 8% after sling operation. The frequency of postoperative de novo urgency after retropubic suspension and sling operation is a little more than that after transvaginal suspension. The use of absorbents and devices are reasonable treatments for female stress incontinence in the short term but are not ideal in the long term.

Key Words. Female stress incontinence, Pelvic floor muscle exercise, α-Adrenergic receptor stimulant, Retropubic suspension, Sling operation

[1] Department of Urology, Shinshu University School of Medicine, 3-1-1 Asahi, Matsumoto 390-8621, Japan
[2] Department of Urology, Nagoya University School of Medicine, 65 Tsurumai, Showa-ku, Nagoya 466-8560, Japan
[3] Department of Obstetrics and Gynecology, Tokyo Metropolitan Police Hospital, 2-10-41 Fujimi, Chiyoda-ku, Tokyo 102-8161, Japan

Introduction

Stress incontinence is a quality of life (QOL) disease, and its severity and the necessity for treatment greatly depend on a patient's individual values. Therefore, in selection of the treatment modality, the patient's own wishes should be considered in addition to efficacy, side effects, invasiveness, and economy. The International Consultation on Incontinence-Questionnaire (ICI-Q) score (Fig. 1) is recommended to assess symptoms of incontinence and their impact on QOL.

---

1   How often do you leak urine? (Tick one box)

never	☐	0
about once a week or less often	☐	1
two or three times a week	☐	2
about once a day	☐	3
several times a day	☐	4
all the time	☐	5

---

2   We would like to know how much urine <u>you think</u> leaks.
How much urine do you <u>usually</u> leak (whether you wear protection or not)?
(Tick one box)

none	☐	0
a small amount	☐	2
a moderate amount	☐	4
a large amount	☐	6

---

3   Overall, how much does leaking urine interfere with your everyday life?

Please ring a number between 0 (not at all) and 10 (a great deal)

     0   1   2   3   4   5   6   7   8   9   **10**

  not at all   a great deal

ICI-Q score: sum scores 3+4+5   [   ]

---

4   When does urine leak? (Please tick all that apply to you)

never - urine does not leak	☐
leaks before you can get to the toilet	☐
leaks when you cough or sneeze	☐
leaks when you are asleep	☐
leaks when you are physically active/exercising	☐
leaks when you have finished urinating and are dressed	☐
leaks for no ovbious reason	☐
leaks all the time	☐

Fɪɢ. 1. International Consultation on Incontinence-Questionnaire (ICI-Q) score

The treatment modalities for female stress incontinence include physiotherapy, drug therapy, surgical treatment, and the use of absorbents and devices.

Physiotherapy

Major physiotherapy for female stress incontinence includes pelvic floor muscle exercise, bladder exercise, electrical stimulation of the pelvic floor muscles, and advice on daily life. Each of these methods is used alone or in combination. Although physiotherapy is the first-line treatment for stress incontinence at present, there are no reports of investigations on how to properly use surgical treatment or noninvasive treatment such as physiotherapy according to severity. Moreover, in Japan the therapeutic procedures described below have the problems that the NHI point of physiotherapy for incontinence has not been established, and some medical equipment necessary for the treatment has not been approved.

Pelvic Floor Muscle Exercise

In the pelvic floor muscle exercise, the levator ani muscle and the periurethral and perivaginal sphincters are voluntarily constricted. It is also called pelvic floor reeducation or pelvic floor rehabilitation [1]. The pelvic floor muscle exercise has the goals of learning how to constrict the urethral sphincter reflexively under the load of abdominal pressure, and increasing urethral closure pressure by strengthening the muscles of the pelvic floor. This exercise is used in a patient who has the ability to understand the purpose of the exercise and who can continue the exercise.

The mechanism (anatomy and physiology) of stress incontinence is first explained to the patient to help her understand the exercise. In exercise, verbal explanation alone is insufficient [2]. The instructor makes the patient recognize the position of the pelvic floor muscles through vaginal examination and teaches her the correct constriction method (manual teaching method). In the basic exercise program, maximum constriction is maintained for 8–12 s, and subsequently the muscle is relaxed for the same period. These procedures are repeated 80–100 times daily. If necessary, the duration and frequency of muscle constriction may be decreased, depending on the patient's muscle power at the start of the exercise. Moreover, the patient is instructed to contract the pelvic floor intentionally when incontinence-inducing stress (for example, coughing, sneezing, or exercise) is applied. As a supportive method to further increase the effect of the pelvic floor muscle exercise, there are periodic intensive exercises by the instructor [3], biofeedback therapy [4], and use of the vaginal cone [5].

In the intensive exercise by the instructor, the patient who has mastered the pelvic floor muscle exercise method visits the rehabilitation center periodically and performs the exercise for a specified period of time. The instructor leads the patient to maximally contract the pelvic floor in various body positions and motivates the patient to continue the same exercise at home. In biofeedback therapy the exercise is performed using equipment that electrically or dynamically monitors constriction of the pelvic floor muscles, by which the patient can perceive the constriction visually and acoustically. Typical equipment includes a vaginal manometer and a electromyogram derived from an electrode on or in the vagina or anus. Recently, several systems that display information from the electromyograph on a personal computer and guide exercise have been commercialized. However, these systems have not been approved by the Ministry of Health, Labor, and Welfare of Japan. There is a useful method that helps the patient understand how to constrict the muscle by confirming the movement of a cylinder of minute diameter inserted in the vagina on constriction of the pelvic floor muscles. A vaginal cone is a weight in the form of a tampon. It is inserted in the vagina, and the patient walks with the pelvic floor muscles constricted so as not to drop the cone. The usual walking time is 15 minutes. There are several grades of weight from 20–100g for cones with the same shape. A patient can select a certain grade of weight according to the muscle power of her pelvic floor.

Pelvic floor muscle exercise was useful as a noninvasive treatment for stress incontinence and produced a significant improvement in a randomized controlled trial (RCT) compared with the group without treatment [6]. In a RCT, in comparison with a group receiving combined pelvic floor muscle exercise and medication (phenylpropanolamine HCl), the group receiving pelvic floor muscle exercise alone showed similar improvement after 6 months of treatment, and there was no difference between the groups [7]. There are few reports on the criteria for application of pelvic floor muscle exercise according to the severity of stress incontinence or patient inconvenience [8]. As a rule, all patients who understand and intend to continue the exercise should be treated by this modality.

When intensive pelvic floor muscle exercise was introduced by the instructor, incontinence significantly improved both subjectively and objectively 6 months later, compared with the group trained at home alone, although no difference was observed between the groups in improvement after the first month. Moreover, when supportive therapy by the biofeedback method is added to the pelvic floor muscle exercise, a more effective result is obtained than with the pelvic floor muscle exercise alone [4,6,9]. The vaginal cone is often used together with pelvic floor muscle exercise, and it improves incontinence when used above. However, pelvic muscle constriction under the guidance of the instructor is significantly more effective than therapy with the vaginal cone only [10].

Bladder Exercise

There are few reports on bladder exercise alone among patients with stress incontinence. In a population with stress incontinence, the frequency of incontinence decreased in those with urge incontinence and those with mixed-type incontinence [11].

Electrical Stimulation of the Pelvic Floor Muscles

Electrical stimulation of the pelvic floor muscles constricts the levator ani muscle and the urethral and anal sphincters at the stimulated sites. Transvaginal, transanal, and percutaneous electrodes are marketed for different routes of electrical stimulation. Although selection of an electrode and treatment schedule (stimulation frequency, frequency of stimulation, frequency of treatment, etc.) have been described in several reports, electrical stimulation is generally provided at 20–50 Hz, two or three times daily for 4–8 weeks for stress incontinence to strengthen the closing function of the external urethral sphincter [12,13]. Vaginal and anal discomfort and pain have been reported, but these effects were not serious. Electrical stimulation is contraindicated in pregnant or possibly pregnant women; women with vaginitis, vaginal fistula, or prolapsed uterus; women with cardiac pacemakers; and women with arrhythmia. An electrical stimulation generator to be used for this treatment has not been approved by the Ministry of Health, Labor, and Welfare of Japan.

Electrical pelvic floor muscle stimulation has not always had significantly favorable results, although improvement in incontinence was observed in a RCT in patients who used sham electrodes [12,14–16]. On the other hand, in a RCT including a group who received electrical stimulation plus pelvic floor muscle exercise, a group who used the vaginal cone, and a group without treatment, pelvic floor muscle exercise alone produced a significant improvement [10]. In patients using both pelvic floor muscle exercise and electrical stimulation therapy, the frequency of incontinence was significantly decreased as compared with patients using sham electrodes [17].

Guidance in Daily Life

Obesity, constipation, smoking, and excessive water intake are risk factors for stress incontinence, and patients are counseled to reduce these factors. Medications are also risk factors. Passive defense methods against stress incontinence include various types of absorptive pads. However, except for unavoidable cases, patients should not be instructed to use such pads during the evaluation period before the start of treatment or until a therapeutic effect is observed.

Drug Therapy

α-Adrenergic Receptor Stimulants

Many α-adrenergic receptors are distributed in the bladder base, bladder neck, and proximal urethra, and α-adrenergic receptor stimulants enhance constriction of the urethral sphincter. Therefore, when an α-adrenergic receptor stimulant is properly administered to a patient with stress incontinence related to intrinsic sphincter deficiency (ISD), it might improve stress incontinence by increasing outflow resistance.

According to this concept, phenylpropanolamine or adrenaline agoniss (ephedrine analogues) have been used for treatment of stress incontinence for a long time. No α-adrenergic receptor stimulant has been registered in the NHI product list for stress incontinence in Japan, but various adrenergic agonists have been marketed on for asthma and orthostatic hypotension, and these drugs may sometimes be used for patients without circulatory complications. However, in a recent clinical study that measured intraurethral pressure, midodrine hydrochloride, a potent α_1-adrenergic receptor stimulant, produced subjective improvement of stress incontinence, but significant changes in maximum urethral closure pressure were not observed [18].

Estrogen Replacement Therapy

Estrogen increases outflow resistance. In postmenopausal women with shrunken urogenitals, estrogen replacement therapy improves the nourishment of the urethral mucous membrane, and increases the thickness of the urethral wall. If estrogen enhances sensitivity to α-adrenergic receptor stimulation, then urethral closure would be improved.

According to a meta-analysis of six reports of estrogen replacement therapy in postmenopausal women with incontinence, subjective improvement occurred in total incontinence and stress incontinence alone. On the other hand, according to objective assessment, leaked urine volume did not decrease in either of these analyses, and only one of six reports showed significant elevation of the maximum urethral closure pressure [19]. In a randomized controlled study in patients with incontinence, estrogen replacement therapy was not effective, as measured by frequency and volume of urine leakage and the results of the pad test [20,21]. However, the urge to micturate and urethral or vaginal infection are often observed in addition to incontinence in postmenopausal women. Estrogen replacement therapy may not improve incontinence itself, but it may relieve subjective problems related to the urethral tract and periurethal sites. Therefore, estrogen replacement therapy should be positioned at present as a secondary therapy for postmenopausal women with incontinence.

Estrogen replacement therapy may be administered by the oral, transvaginal, and percutaneous routes. At present, injection cannot be used for long-term estrogen replacement. Oral estrogen preparations now on the market include conjugated estrogen (CEE) and estriol (E3), the percutaneous preparation is estradiol (E2), and the transvaginal preparation is E3. In patients receiving estrogen therapy for incontinence, oral CEE 0.3–1.25 mg/day has often been administered experimentally as a part of estrogen replacement therapy for other purposes, including prevention of climacteric disturbance or arteriosclerosis and management of osteoporosis. However, this dosage is based on investigations in Europe and North America. It will be necessary to determine optimal dosages for Japanese women, who have ethnic differences and smaller physiques. To prevent endometrial carcinoma, parallel periodic or repeated administration of progestin preparations such as medroxyprogesterone acetate (MPA) is recommended when estrogen is administered at this dose for a long period. For periodic administration, MPA at doses of 2.5–10 mg/day per cycle (4 weeks to 1 month) is administered for 12–15 days. For repeated administration, MPA at doses of 2.5–10 mg/day is administered every day.

E3 is often used for the treatment of vaginal atrophy by the oral and transvaginal routes in Japan because of its small effect on the endometrium. However, oral administration of E3 at a dose of 3 mg/day did not produce significant subjective or objective therapeutic effects on de novo urgency or irritative symptoms of the lower urinary tract [22]. Percutaneous administration of E2 is a relatively new estrogen replacement therapy, and it has the advantages of little effect on the liver and relatively lower blood E2 level. Two or more formulations have been marketed in Japan. When the standard dose of estrogen replacement therapy is used in climacteric women, parallel administration of progestin should be considered. If a dose of E2 that sufficiently relieves climacteric symptoms is administered percutaneously, it also has therapeutic effects on complaints related to the lower urethral tract, such as de novo urgency, but the optimal percutaneous dose of E2 has not been established. There is no reasonable basis to recommend the parallel administration of progestin to women undergoing uterectomy, because it has not yet been clarified whether the occurrence of breast cancer is inhibited by progestin replacement.

Estrogen replacement therapy has preventive effects against cerebrovascular disorders, ischemic cardiac disease, and osteoporosis, in addition to improving urinary disturbance. However, in patients with hysteromyoma, endometriosis, endometrial hyperplasia with cellular atypia, or mastopathy with cellular atypia, estrogen replacement therapy is disadvantageous. In patients who have endometrial carcinoma or breast cancer or who have recently had these diseases, estrogen replacement therapy is inappropriate. Therapeutic procedures other than estrogen replacement therapy should be used to treat incontinence in patients with these conditions.

β-Adrenergic Receptor Stimulant

Clenbuterol hydrochloride, a β-adrenergic receptor stimulant, has been used as an antasthmatic for a long time. It has been listed in NHI products for treatment of stress incontinence. It is thought that a β-receptor stimulant increases outflow resistance at the bladder neck by increasing muscle tone of the striated muscles of the pelvic floor. After 2 weeks of repeated administration of clenbuterol hydrochloride at a daily dose of 20–40 μg in 32 patients with stress incontinence, the rate of effectiveness, including remarkable and moderate improvements in frequency and volume of urine leakage, was 75%; adverse effects, including tremor and palpitation, were observed in 32% of patients [23]. Two other clinical studies showed that clenbuterol hydrochloride decreased the frequency and volume of urine leakage after oral administration at a dose of 20–40 μg/day [24,25].

The therapeutic effects of clenbuterol hydrochloride are comparable to those of pelvic floor muscle exercise, but the usefulness of clenbuterol hydrochloride does not exceed that of pelvic floor muscle exercise with regard to cost, frequency of hospital visits, and adverse effects. Furthermore, when these therapeutic results are compared with those of surgical treatment over a long period of time, clenbuterol hydrochloride is inferior to surgery in therapeutic effect, cost, frequency of hospital visits, and adverse effects. Therefore, management by clenbuterol hydrochloride is a convenient method, but it is difficult to conclude that the method has an advantage in long-term management of stress incontinence. However, because it does not require special equipment for diagnosis or treatment and the patient can be restored to be original condition any time, treatment with clenbuterol hydrochloride has advantages over surgical treatment. Clenbuterol hydrochloride increases blood pressure and blood glucose and therefore is not appropriate for hypertensive and diabetic patients.

Surgical Treatment

When surgical treatment for female stress incontinence is selected, investigation of the etiologic factors of stress incontinence, that is, evaluation of hypermobility of the bladder neck and intrinsic sphincter deficiency (ISD) and investigation of detrusor instability (DI), by objective examinations is required, including urodynamic examination and cystography in addition to examination of subjective symptoms. Various operative techniques and their modifications have been performed. They can be classified into five categories: retropubic suspension, transvaginal suspension, sling operation, anterior repair, and periurethral injection of bulking agents.

Retropubic and transvaginal suspension aim to support or suspend the bladder neck from the proximal urethra and to prevent its descent. They are performed in the patient who has normal sphincter function and hypermobility of the bladder neck. The sling operation aims at coaptation of the proximal urethra-bladder neck in ISD in addition to preventing descent of the bladder neck, and is used in patients who have intrinsic sphincter deficiency or bladder neck hypermobility. Periurethral injection of bulking agents aims at coaptation of the proximal urethra-bladder neck, and as a rule it is used in patients with intrinsic sphincter deficiency.

Comparison of the clinical results between various types of techniques is not easy, because definition of the improvement of incontinence varies among published reports, few reports have studied the long-term effects, the operative techniques are not consistent and are often modified by surgeons, and there are very few reports of randomized comparative studies. The following surgical results are mainly based on the meta-analytical results of a long-term study [26] that was performed under the guidelines for surgical treatment of female stress incontinence prepared by the American Urological Association in 1997 (Clinical Practice Guideline) and the results of recent randomized comparative studies. Meta-analytical results of a long-term study (4 year or more) showed that the elimination rates of incontinence (median values) were 84% for retropubic suspension, 67% for transvaginal suspension, 83% for sling operation, and 61% for anterior repair, and consequently retropubic suspension and sling operation were more effective than the other surgical techniques.

Major complications of surgical operations for incontinence include urinary disturbance due to urethral obstruction and postoperative de novo urgency. Meta-analytical results suggest that the frequency of transient urinary retention for 4 weeks or more was about 5% after transvaginal suspension and about 8% after the sling operation [26]. There are not sufficient data on the frequency of permanent urinary retention for analysis. The frequency of postoperative de novo urgency after retropubic suspension and sling operation was a little higher than after transvaginal suspension [26]. No differences between surgical techniques are observed in complications related to urinary tract infection or wound infection, whereas complications of vaginal erosion, urethral erosion, fistula, or wound infection were more frequent in the group of patients who underwent the sling operation with a sling of artificial material than in those who had a sling made of vital tissue.

Retropubic Suspension

Retropubic suspension aims to suspend or support periurethral/bladder neck tissue using Cooper's ligament or the pubic periosteum as an anchor after lower abdominal section. Typical technique includes the Marshall-Marchetti-Kranz method, in which the peritissue of the urethra/bladder neck and retropubic periosteum are sutured, and Burch's method, in which Cooper's ligament is sutured, which is applied in patients with bladder neck hypermobility. With recent trends toward less invasive treatment and the development of laparoscopic techniques, the usefulness of Burch's technique with a laparoscope has been studied. The results of Burch's surgical technique with a laparoscope are now under evaluation [27,28], and consequently the long-term results are unknown.

Transvaginal Suspension

Transvaginal suspension includes Stamey's method, Gittes' method, and Raz's method. In Japan, Stamey's method has been widely used since the mid-1980s. It is applied to patients with bladder neck hypermobility. Transvaginal suspension had good short-term results but poor long-term results [29]. Recently, the sling operation has been selected even for patients with bladder neck hypermobility [30]. In patients who have intrinsic sphincter deficiency and bladder neck hypermobility, the improvement rate is poor [31]. The short-term clinical results were equivalent to those with Burch's retropubic suspension [32,33], whereas the long-term results were inferior [26], although it is difficult to compare the results of different techniques. Furthermore, the results of transvaginal suspension in patients with intrinsic sphincter deficiency were inferior to the results in patients with bladder neck hypermobility [31].

Sling Operation of Bladder Neck (Urethra)

There are transabdominal and transvaginal techniques, and the less invasive transvaginal sling operation is popular for female stress incontinence. It is applied to patients with intrinsic sphincter deficiency or to patients in whom other operations for incontinence have failed. Recently, it has also been applied to patients with bladder neck hypermobility [27]. Vital tissue such as fascia (fascia of rectus abdominis muscle, tensor of femoral fascia, vaginal wall) or synthetic material such as Marlex mesh and Gore-Tex are used as material for the sling. The long-term results are good, but there are problems of postoperative lower urethral occlusion or de novo urgency. In recent years, the technique without the application of tension to the sling (no-tension sling) has been popular, based on the idea not to suspend but to support the bladder neck or urethra with the sling. The tension-free vaginal tape (TVT) sling operation, which supports the center of the urethra with proline tape as a sling, is used as a less invasive technique that can be done under local anesthesia. Both the short-term and the long-term results of the sling operation showed stably desirable results in the elimination rate of incontinence regardless of the pathologic condition of incontinence. Although there are few reports of the TVT sling, the short-term results with the use of the TVT sling in a large-scale, randomized study were equivalent to the results with Burch's surgical technique [34], and the results of a long-term study showed that the elimination rate of incontinence was 91%, an excellent result [35].

Anterior Repair

The elimination rate of incontinence with anterior repair was poor compared with Burch's retropubic suspension in both short-term and long-term studies [36,37].

Periurethral Injection of Bulking Agents

GAX collagen is injected under the bladder neck/proximal urethra mucous membrane for coaptation of the bladder neck-proximal urethra. Periurethral injection of bulking agents is used in patients with intrinsic sphincter deficiency. Injection is performed by needle puncture under transurethral endoscope or by the periurethral route. It has a high recurrence rate, and often needs two or more repeated injections to obtain stable efficacy. In periurethral injection of bulking agents, the recurrence rate is high, the rate of elimination of incontinence is lower than with the other surgical techniques, and the long-term results are unknown.

Absorbents and Devices

Absorbents (pads and diapers) of various forms to absorb the leaked urine are widely used to manage incontinence. Recently, skin troubles related to the use of absorbents have been greatly reduced by technical developments. Pads and diapers can be easily used without anxiety and without the help of medical staff, and they are easily available, except for special products. Moreover, data related to micturition, such as recording of micturition diary and measurement of urine leakage, can be generated by using the absorbent for an indicated period of time.

However, permanent use of the absorbent is a problem. Even if a patient can participate in social activities by using a pad or diaper, she still feels she has a physical defect. QOL is decreased by the need to bring absorbents to work and the interference with leisure activities such as sports and travel. Many patients with stress incontinence are eligible for surgical treatment. The expenses of management with pad or diaper would exceed the expenses of surgical treatment in a few years.

The device, which is a little different from the absorbent, includes a pessary that is inserted in the vagina to support the bladder neck, a lid that covers the external urethra, and a urethral plug that is inserted in the urethra. Although the device is similar to the absorbent in that it does not improve the physical condition causing urine leakage, it differs from absorbent in that the device is intended to decrease involuntary urine leakage. The rate of elimination of stress incontinence with the urethral plug was about 38% in two reports [38,39], and the adverse effects of urinary tract infection and accidental drop of an urethral plug in the bladder were observed. If convenience is considered, the clinical results with the urethral plug are favorable. However, the urethral plug has been marketed in few contries, and there is no plan to submit an application for approval to market the product in Japan. A pessary that is inserted in the vagina to support the bladder neck was marketed for a while in Japan, but there is no plan for commercial marketing in the future, and the prospects for evaluation of the clinical results are still far from certain. The absorbent and device are reasonable treatment modalities for female stress incontinence on a short-time basis but not for long periods.

References

1. Kegel AH (1948) Progressive exercise in the functional restoration of the perineal muscles. Am J Obstet Gynecol 56:238–248
2. Bump RC, Hurt WG, Fantl JA, Wyman JF (1991) Assessment of Kegel pelvic muscle exercise performance after brief verbal instruction. Am J Obstet Gynecol 165:322–327
3. Bo K, Hagen RM, Kvarstein B, Jorgensen J, Larsen S (1990) Pelvic floor muscle exercises for the treatment of female stress urinary incontinence III. Effects of two different degrees of pelvic floor muscle exercises. Neurourol Urodyn 9:489–502
4. Burgio KL, Robinson JC, Engel BT (1986) The role of biofeedback in Kegel exercise training for stress urinary incontinence. Am J Obstet Gynecol 154:58–64
5. Wilson PD, Borland M (1990) Vaginal cones for the treatment of genuine stress incontinence. Aust N Z J Obstet Gynaecol 30:157–160
6. Burns PA, Pranikoff K, Nochajski TH, Hadley EC, Levy KJ, Ory MG (1993) A comparison of effectiveness of biofeedback and pelvic muscle excercise treatment of stress incontinence in older community-dwelling women. J Gerontol 48:M167–M174
7. Wells TJ, Brink CA, Diokno AC, Wolfe R, Gillis GL (1991) Pelvic muscle exercise for stress urinary incontinence in elderly women. J Am Geriatr Soc 39:785–791

8. Elia G, Bergman A (1993) Pelvic muscle exercises: when do they work? Obstet Gynecol 81:283–286m

9. Glavind K, Nohr SB, Walter S (1996) Biofeedback and physiotherapy versus physiotherapy alone in the treatment of genuine stress urinary incontinence. Int Urogynecol 7:339–343

10. Bo K, Talseth T, Holme I (1999) Single blind, randomised controlled trial of pelvic floor exercises, electrical stimulation, vaginal cones, and no treatment in management of genuine stress incontinence. BMJ 318:487–493

11. Fantl JA, Wyman JF, McClish DK, Hrkins SW, Elswick RK, Taylor JR, Hadley EC (1991) Efficacy of bladder training in older women with urinary incontinence. JAMA 265:609–613

12. Sand PK, Richardson DA, Staskin DR, Swift SE, Appell RA, Whitmore KE, Ostergard DR (1995) Pelvic floor electrical stimulation in the treatment of genuine stress incontinence: a multicenter, placebo-controlled trial. Am J Obstet Gynecol 173:72–79

13. Luber KM, Wolde-Tsadik G (1997) Efficacy of functional electrical stimulation in treating genuine stress incontinence: a randomized clinical trial. Neurourol Urodyn 16:543–551

14. Yamanishi T, Yasuda K, Sakakibara R, Hattori T, Ito H, Murakami S (1997) Pelvic floor electrical stimulation in the treatment of stress incontinence: an investigational study and a placebo controlled double-blind trial. J Urol 158:2127–2131

15. Luber KM, Wolde-Tsadik G (1997) Efficacy of functional electrical stimulation in treating genuine stress incontinence: a randomized clinical trial. Neurourol Urodyn 16:543–551

16. Laycock J, Jerwood D (1993) Does pre-modulated interferential therapy cure genuine stress incontinence? Physiotherapy 79:553–560

17. Blowman C, Pickles C, Emery S, Creates V, Towell L, Blackburn N, Doyle N, Walkden B (1991) Prospective double blind controlled trial of intensive physiotherapy with and without stimulation of the pelvic floor in treatment of genuine stress incontinence. Physiotherapy 77:661–664

18. Weil EH, Eerdmans PH, Dijkman GA, Tamussino K, Feyereisl J, Vierhout ME, Schmidbauer C, Egarter C, Kolle D, Plasman JE, Heidler H, Abbuhl BE, Wein W (1998) Randomized double-blind placebo-controlled multicenter evaluation of efficacy and dose finding of midodrine hydrochloride in women with mild to moderate stress urinary incontinence: a phase II study. Int Urogynecol J Pelvic Floor Dysfunct 9:145–150

19. Fantl JA, Cardozo L, McClish DK (1994) Estrogen therapy in the management of urinary incontinence in postmenopausal women: a meta-analysis. First report of the Hormones and Urogenital Therapy Committee. Obstet Gynecol 83:12–18

20. Fantl JA, Bump RC, Robinson D, McClish DK, Wyman JF (1996) Efficacy of estrogen supplementation in the treatment of urinary incontinence. The Continence Program for Women Research Group. Obstet Gynecol 88:745–749

21. Jackson S, Shepherd A, Brookes S, Abrams P (1999) The effect of oestrogen supplementation on post-menopausal urinary stress incontinence: a double-blind placebo-controlled trial. Br J Obstet Gynaecol 106:711–718

22. Cardozo L, Rekers H, Tapp A, Barnick C, Shepherd A, Schussler B, Kerr-Wilson R, van Geelan J, Barlebo H, Walter S (1993) Oestriol in the treatment of postmenopausal urgency: a multicentre study. Maturitas 18:47–53

23. Shimazaki J, Yasuda K, Yamanishi T, et al. (1995) A clinical trial of clenbuterol granule in stress incontinence. Jpn Pharmacol Ther 23:3379–3395

24. Shimazaki J, Yasuda K, Imabayashi K, et al. (1992) Dose finding study on clenbuterol in stress incontinence. Jpn J Urol Surg 5:933–945

25. Kawabe K, Kageyama S, Honma Y, et al. (1995) A clinical trial of clenbuterol granule in stress incontinence. Jpn Pharmacol Ther 23:3361–3377

26. Leach GE, Dmochowski RR, Appell RA, Blaivas JG, Hadley HR, Luber KM, Mostwin JL, O'Donnell PD, Roehrborn CG (1997) Female stress urinary incontinence clinical guidelines panel summary report on surgical management of female stress urinary incontinence. J Urol 158:875–880

27. Burton B (1997) A three year prospective randomized urodynamic study comparing open and laparoscopic colposuspension. Neurourol Urodyn 16:353–357

28. Ross J (1996) Two techniques of laparoscopic Burch repair for stress incontinence: a prospective, randomized study. J Am Assoc Gynecol Laparosc 3:351–357

29. Conrad S, Pieper A, Fernandez S, Bush R, Huland H (1997) Long-term results of the Stamey bladder neck suspension procedure; a patient questionnaire based outcome analysis. J Urol 157:1672–1677

30. Chaikin DC, Rosenthal J, Blaivas JG (1998) Pubovaginal fascial sling for all types of stress urinary incontinence: long-term analysis. J Urol 160:1312–1316

31. Kondo A, Kato K, Gotoh M, Narushima M, Saito M (1998) The Stamey and Gittes procedures: long-term followup in relation to incontinence types and patient age. J Urol 160:756–758

32. Gilja I, Puskar D, Mazuran B, Radej M (1998) Comparative analysis of bladder neck suspension using Raz, Burch and transvaginal Burch procedures: a 3-year randomized prospective study. Eur Urol 33:298–302

33. Athanassopoulos A, Barbalias G (1996) Burch colposuspension versus Stamey endoscopic bladder neck suspension: a urodynamic appraisal. Urol Int 56:23–27

34. Ward KL, Hilton P, Browning J (2000) A randomized trial of colposuspension and tension-free vaginal tape (TVT) for primary genuine stress incontinence. Neurourol Urodynam 19:386–387

35. Ulmsten U, Johnson P, Rezapour M (1999) A three-years followup of tension free vaginal tape for surgical treatment of female stress urinary incontinence. Br J Obstet Gynecol 106:345–350

36. Kammerer-Doak DN, Dorin MH, Rogers RG, Cousin MO (1999) A randomized trial of Burch retropubic urethropexy and anterior corporrhaphy for stress urinary incontinence. Obstet Gynecol 93:75–78

37. Liapis A, Pyrgiotis E, Kontoravdis A, Louridas C, Zourlas PA (1996) Genuine stress incontinence: prospective randomized comparison of two operative methods. Eur J Obstet Gynecol Reprod Biol 64:69–72

38. Nielsen KK, Walter S, Maegaard E, Kromann-Andersen B (1995) The urethral plug— an alternative treatment of women with urinary stress incontinence. Ugeskr Laeger 157:3194–3197

39. Sand PK, Staskin D, Miller J, Sant GR, Davila GW, Knapp P, Rappaport S, Tutrone R (1999) Effect of a urinary control insert on quality of life in incontinent women. Int Urogynecol J Pelvic Floor Dysfunct 10:100–105

Subject Index